OUR BEACHES WERE EMPTY, OUR HOSPITALS FULL

Leadership Stories from Hawai‘i's
Unique Pandemic Response

OUR BEACHES WERE EMPTY, OUR HOSPITALS FULL

Leadership Stories from Hawai‘i’s Unique Pandemic Response

Kirk Caldwell
and
Georgette Takushi Deemer

LEGACY ISLE
PUBLISHING

ISBN 978-1-958701-02-7

Library of Congress Control Number: 2023901172

Design and production
Ingrid Lynch

Cover photography
© Ric Noyle

Legacy Isle Publishing
1000 Bishop St., Ste. 806
Honolulu, HI 96813
Telephone 1-808-587-7766
Toll-free 1-866-900-BOOK
www.legacyislepublishing.net
info@legacyislepublishing.net

Printed in Korea

Contents

Introduction 7

The Contributors 10

CHAPTER 1
When Did You Know and What Did You Do? 15

CHAPTER 2
Lockdown 60

CHAPTER 3
Health vs. Business 106

CHAPTER 4
The Dreaded Second Surge 149

CHAPTER 5
Tiers and Fears 176

CHAPTER 6
Hope in a Vaccine 207

CHAPTER 7
Lessons Learned 224

CHAPTER 8
Through an Aspirational Lens 258

EPILOGUE
Where Do We Go from Here? 309

Introduction

People have asked why we'd want to write a book about the COVID-19 pandemic in Hawai'i. Everyone, including us, would like to forget about it—put it behind us and get on with our lives.

We understand the need for Hawai'i's people to move forward and not dwell on the past. Yet, it would be unfortunate for us as a community not to record what happened in Hawai'i as COVID-19 reached our shores.

As far as we know, no book has been written about how the people of Hawai'i addressed the last worldwide pandemic, the Spanish flu of 1918–1919. We wish there were such a book. It could have provided a valuable resource for actions to take, and what worked and what did not. It would have helped us understand how the community would respond and how businesses would be impacted. It would have provided insight on how decisions were made and by whom.

There's another good reason for writing *Our Beaches Were Empty, Our Hospitals Full.* It is important to write our history—to tell our stories, particularly when they revolve around significant and extraordinary times in our state, our country, and the world. We wanted to preserve a record of what happened and why.

This book tells the story of Hawai'i's response to the pandemic by those who were on the front lines in the battle against COVID-19. There were many Island leaders who were critical to the effort, and for this book we chose to interview the top decision maker in each organization or company represented here. They were the ones who had to stand behind their decisions and be held accountable. You will hear their stories in detail as they recount their responses to the pandemic.

One thing that becomes evident from these interviews is that none of these leaders had a playbook to turn to in the event of such a pandemic. All of them put teams in place to advise them on actions to be taken to protect their organizations and the people they served.

There was a sharing of information among some of these organizations that led to critical decisions to slow the spread of the virus and reopen our community and economy in a safe manner. This sharing of information was enhanced by the Hawai'i Executive Collaborative (HEC), an integral network of private and public sector entities organized by Island business leader Duane Kurisu a couple of years before the pandemic struck our shores. This organization stepped to the forefront of decision-making during the pandemic and provided valuable assistance to the State of Hawai'i, the City and County of Honolulu, other government organizations, and both for-profit and nonprofit businesses.

Never before in Hawai'i, we believe, had there been such an open and honest discussion among competing institutions in such a collaborative style. This represents the core values of who we are as a community. The work of the HEC shows us at our very best, as a people who practice aloha and embrace our *kuleana*, our responsibility, even in the worst of times.

During the first year of the pandemic, 2020, we worked intimately with Hawai'i's various communities and their leaders. For this book, we identified and interviewed twenty-five of those leaders representing government agencies, medical organizations and hospitals, doctors on the mayor's COVID-19 advisory panel, business and nonprofit organizations, banks, and public and private educational institutions. By no account is this an exhaustive list. There are countless leaders who worked tirelessly to help Hawai'i fight the disease and protect our population. Every one of them are heroes.

All of the interviews for this book were recorded in 2021. Therefore, readers should note that certain things may have changed or evolved since that time. The book is essentially a compilation of those firsthand interviews organized by the chronological progression of COVID-19 as we all endured the catastrophic events of 2020. When we first began planning this story of Hawai'i's pandemic response we expected that a vaccine would become available toward the end of the year and that the vaccine would be the tool we needed to bring the pandemic under control. We anticipated that, in 2021 and beyond, COVID-19 might still be with us but well managed, with Hawai‘i in full recovery mode.

As we now know, that did not happen. As we worked on the book, Hawai‘i continued to wrestle with record case counts due to new variants while we witnessed a society split between the vaccinated and unvaccinated, businesses that were unable to hold on, and, overall, a weary community. Yet, the spirit of Hawai‘i is resilient.

Which leads to a final point. What will remain forever in our minds and hearts is the incredible sacrifice and effort made by the people of Hawai‘i during this crisis. The extraordinary amount of compassion, cooperation, and, most of all, perseverance shown by our community is nothing short of a miracle. We should all be so very proud of our collective actions. ❋

The Contributors

We thank the following leaders who were interviewed for this book, and who generously shared their time, stories, and manaʻo.

Chris Benjamin, President and Chief Executive Officer, Alexander & Baldwin

Elizabeth (Libby) Char, MD, Director, State of Hawaiʻi Department of Health (prior to September 2020: Medical Director, Honolulu Fire Department)

Timothy Cottrell, Head of School, ʻIolani School

David Derauf, MD, Executive Director, Kōkua Kalihi Valley

John De Fries, President and Chief Executive Officer, Hawaiʻi Tourism Authority

Jonathan Dworkin, MD, The Queen's Medical Center, Internal Medicine and Infectious Disease

Dennis Francis, President and Publisher, Oahu Publications (*The Honolulu Star-Advertiser*)

Bob Harrison, Chairman of the Board, President and Chief Executive Officer, First Hawaiian Bank

Jason Higa, Chief Executive Officer, FCH Enterprises (parent company of Zippy's restaurants)

Peter Ho, Chairman, President and Chief Executive Officer, Bank of Hawai'i

David Ige, Governor of Hawai'i, 2014–2022

Peter Ingram, President and Chief Executive Officer, Hawaiian Airlines and parent company Hawaiian Holdings

Micah Kane, Chief Executive Officer and President, Hawai'i Community Foundation

Derek Kawakami, Mayor, County of Kaua'i

Harry Kim, Mayor, County of Hawai'i, 2016–2020

Christina Kishimoto, Superintendent, State of Hawai'i Department of Education, 2017–2021

Duane Kurisu, Chairman, Chief Executive Officer and Owner, aio, LLC; Chairman, Hawai'i Executive Collaborative

David Lassner, President, University of Hawai'i

Sherry Menor-McNamara, Chief Executive Officer, Chamber of Commerce Hawai'i

Ron Mizutani, President and Chief Executive Officer, Hawai'i Foodbank, 2018–2021

Mark Mugiishi, President and Chief Executive Officer, HMSA (Hawaii Medical Service Association)

Ray Vara, President and Chief Executive Officer, Hawai'i Pacific Health

Michael Victorino, Mayor, County of Maui

Paul Yokota, President, FCH Enterprises, (parent company of Zippy's restaurants)

Paul Yonamine, Chairman and Chief Executive Officer, Central Pacific Financial Corporation

CONTRIBUTORS BY FIELD

Government

Governor David Ige, State of Hawai'i
Mayor Derek Kawakami, County of Kaua'i
Mayor Harry Kim, County of Hawai'i
Mayor Michael Victorino, County of Maui

Healthcare

Dr. Libby Char, State of Hawai'i Department of Health
Dr. David DeRauf, Kōkua Kalihi Valley
Dr. Jonathan Dworkin, The Queen's Health System
Dr. Mark Mugiishi, Hawaii Medical Service Association
Ray Vara, Hawai'i Pacific Health

Business

Chris Benjamin, Alexander & Baldwin
John De Fries, Hawai'i Tourism Authority
Dennis Francis, *The Honolulu Star Advertiser*
Bob Harrison, First Hawaiian Bank
Jason Higa, Zippy's
Peter Ho, Bank of Hawai'i
Peter Ingram, Hawaiian Airlines
Duane Kurisu, aio, LLC

Sherry Menor-McNamara, Chamber of Commerce Hawai‘i
Paul Yokota, Zippy's
Paul Yonamine, Central Pacific Bank

Education

Tim Cottrell, ‘Iolani School
Christina Kishimoto, State of Hawai‘i Department of Education
David Lassner, University of Hawai‘i

Non-Profit Organizations

Micah Kane, Hawai‘i Community Foundation
Ron Mizutani, Hawai‘i Foodbank

INTERVIEWERS

Kirk Caldwell, Mayor, City and County of Honolulu, 2013–2021
Georgette Deemer, Deputy Managing Director, City and County of Honolulu, 2013–2021
Gary Kurokawa, Chief of Staff to the Mayor, City and County of Honolulu, 2016–2021

CHAPTER 1

When Did You Know and What Did You Do?

The first question we asked all the interviewees was "When did you first hear about COVID-19 and what actions did you take, if any?"

In January 2020, Dr. Timothy Cottrell, the head of school at 'Iolani School, one of Honolulu's top independent college preparatory academies, was riding in a car with distinguished alumnus Dr. Vernon Oi, a world-renowned Stanford University immunological researcher who is now retired and living on the Big Island.

Tim Cottrell Vernon is like a godfather of genomics. He's a co-holder of two of the five most valuable patents in the history of Stanford. Vernon was visiting O'ahu and we were driving and listening to NPR (National Public Radio), and they were talking about this thing happening in China—another SARS-related virus. Given Vernon's expertise as an immunological researcher, he shared that the prior two SARS outbreaks were super serious but contained—the one in the Middle East and the one that happened in China. And I didn't think anything of it at the time, but he said right then, "This could be really serious."

This was back in January 2020, before there was a lot of talk about COVID, but I thought, well, this is a little bit like an EF Hutton moment; when this guy says it might be serious, you should listen. He'd been talking to other colleagues and had some insight on how bad it could be. Because of this, we also reached out to 'Iolani School alumnus Dr. Jerome Kim, the director general of the International Vaccine Institute, based in Seoul. He was able to give us immediate real-time updates on the situation globally.

Tim Cottrell had another important concern. 'Iolani had about forty students from China in its boarding program at that time, and some of them were from Wuhan.

Tim Cottrell One boarding student's father was a frontline doctor in China who had been involved in curtailing the first SARS. While we had contacts on the ground, we didn't receive any special insight because there was no flow of information about the virus. All we knew was that it was a serious situation, and some of our students would likely be unable to return home for a while. We immediately started working on plans for their accommodations, planning for a variety of scenarios, including if we had to shut down.

David Lassner, president of the University of Hawai'i, also had an EF Hutton moment while on a site visit at the University of Nebraska Medical School in February.

David Lassner We were in Omaha, Nebraska, for a potential donor visit with a person of wealth who owned a home on the Big Island. This individual and his group had done a lot at the University of Nebraska medical campus, so we toured the Omaha campus to see what they had been able to accomplish in partnership with the university. The chancellor of the University of Nebraska Omaha was also the chancellor of the medical school there. He was an MD who was very engaged in our national response to COVID-19; some of the early cruise ship patients were quarantined in their secure facility. I still remember that nobody was masking at the time, but when I reached out to shake hands he declined and offered me my first elbow bump.

This was mid-February and he basically said if we didn't get this right, half a million Americans were going to die. That was his number. The next day he jetted off to Washington, DC, where he was one of the advisors to the US government. That was my wake-up call. I got back home and found that we were still clear here. But that's when we started talking about our planning and then, as the numbers started growing, we knew we would have to take action.

In downtown Honolulu, Peter Ho, chairman, president, and CEO of *Bank of Hawaiʻi, was thinking about Chinese New Year in January 2020. He remembers brief conversations about something happening in Wuhan.*

Peter Ho I remember asking, "Do you think there's anything here?" And who knew? But what I did know was that the Chinese government had canceled Chinese New Year in China, and in Wuhan in particular, and knowing something about Chinese people, I said, "That's crazy! I mean, these people are clearly frightened." And the more there was this narrative around "there's nothing to worry about," the more I worried about it because I just thought that the two didn't square. The Chinese are incredibly commercial people and if there really wasn't anything to worry about, they wouldn't be worried and they'd be celebrating the most important holiday season of their culture.

In late January, we started having meetings. I looked in my Outlook calendar, which had "meeting on the virus in China." We didn't know about COVID, but we convinced ourselves that it's better to be prepared than not. I think we were one of the first organizations to really start pandemic planning. We wanted a plan to give us the confidence of having a plan in the event that this actually played out in any meaningful way. And, unfortunately, the news just continued to get worse.

What's scary is we have all sorts of plans, but we'd never really gotten around to this because, number one, everyone thought it would be a black swan event. And number two, I think that it had been a hundred years [since the last pandemic]; there's no resource to turn to. *What would you do?* This is thematically one of the very interesting things of the pandemic.

I turned to people I knew who could pull together data conceptually and the closest I could come up with was the Hawaii Data Collaborative, which is Mike Mohr and Pierre Omidyar's group. And, thankfully, Ray Vara, who I'm very close to and who is on our board, was thinking the same thing.

Ray Vara is president and CEO of Hawai'i Pacific Health (HPH). In January 2020, HPH started tracking the virus internally and bringing together some of their physicians for their insights and thoughts. As time went on and the virus started spreading in key cities across the world, Peter knew instinctively that we in Hawai'i had a problem and together with Ray went to the Hawaii Data Collaborative.

Peter Ho You know what's very hard to understand is the power of interest compounding, the power of exponential outcome. Most minds work in a very linear fashion. I just intuitively understood that by the time you realize you have a problem, it's probably already been a problem. And the power of "exponentiality"—that's a real problem. It was the knowledge of how these things compound and the realization that a lot of people don't understand the fury of how things compound.

Ray already had people who could do these calculations, but he needed a third party to help validate that this was not just HPH coming up with this stuff. That third party was the Hawai'i Data Collaborative.

At the City and County of Honolulu, not only was no data being collected, there was no playbook on pandemic planning. Because the City does not have a health department and is reliant on the State of Hawai'i for that function, it turned to the Department of Emergency Management (DEM) for advice on where to start planning for a possible pandemic.

Kirk Caldwell In January, I asked our director of DEM, Hiro Toiya, to find the binder compiled approximately ten years prior on what the City does when there's a pandemic. I got it, sat down with our chief of staff, Gary Kurokawa, and we read through it, just quickly, for about forty-five minutes. There was one page where you check the boxes to see if you have a pandemic or not. We didn't check them all, but we checked most of them, more than 50 percent, and we said, "We've got a pandemic! It's not in Hawai'i, but there's a pandemic and it's spreading."

This binder was not prepared to protect the public health of the residents of O'ahu—that was the Hawai'i State Department of Health's job. It was a primer on how you keep the continuity of your city government functioning if there's a pandemic. How you make sure water continues to flow; your sewers are working; that people are picking up your garbage; that your city workers can come to work and process things to make sure basic city government functions continue to operate such as the police, fire, and EMS. It wasn't about the human health details; for that, no such book existed.

I went on a trip to the continent at the end of January and I took hand sanitizer on the plane—I never did that before, but I was reading that it would be a helpful protective measure. And I wasn't wearing a mask. I thought about it, but they weren't saying you gotta wear a mask yet, so I didn't wear a mask. The plane was packed. I remember asking the flight attendant, local guy, coming back on Delta, "Hey, are you seeing any impact? Hear anything? People not coming, not traveling?" He said, "No, things are good. Look how busy we are! Here, take a whole bunch of cookies, Mayor!"

So when I came back, I had some concern that I had traveled. And then on February 18, I asked Sarah Park, who was the state epidemiologist, to meet with me and the heads of the police department, fire department, emergency management, EMS, the top guys in our administration, and a few other people, and basically Sarah told us we didn't need to be concerned.

She said that wearing masks did not show that they protected you. We were hearing things by then about temperatures checks and she said they were not effective, they didn't necessarily catch someone who had COVID, a higher temperature could be other things. She said it was no worse than the flu and she said the best thing to do was to wash our hands. While we did have a discussion, I felt troubled by her responses. My *na'au* was telling me that more had to be done.

Then we heard about the cases in Washington State in care homes where people were dying. And I started realizing we're human beings—we all have the same DNA and we all get sick together, we all get the flu together. It could come here; it looked like it was having an impact not just in China and in the state of Washington, but other places around the world.

Governor David Ige became aware of the first case of COVID in the United States just before the New Year's holiday.

David Ige I definitely was aware of the impact of SARS and some of the other diseases on Hawai'i's economy. So, it was a concern pretty early on about what we needed to anticipate, what would be happening, and we knew that we had to get in front of it before it got away.

I attended the National Governors Association meeting in DC. It actually was scheduled two weeks earlier than usual, so it was the first weekend in February. The winter meeting is always in DC. Typically, there would be the White House dinner and all of those kinds of things with broad participation by the governors, and because it's in DC it usually ends up being more robust than other conferences.

There were a couple of things added to the agenda because of COVID. And it wasn't really initially planned, but the Department of Homeland Security under the Trump administration had made a special presentation—a classified presentation, because they wanted to keep the discussion frank and private. The federal agencies, particularly the Department of Homeland Security, Federal Emergency Management Association (FEMA), and Department of Health and Human Services, made it pretty clear that they thought this virus was very serious, we needed to take it very seriously, and we needed to take action.

But, obviously, this was Donald Trump. And they also made it clear that the federal government would not be taking the lead on a lot of the initiatives; states should be prepared to respond on their own.

We had made preparations to conduct testing in the state of Hawai'i because we knew with SARS and previous experiences that being able to test locally was going to be very important. We were already sending samples to the CDC (Centers for Disease Control and Prevention) in Atlanta to see if COVID was here. The State has a pretty good surveillance system and doctors are used to taking samples for flu. We were processing them at that time, trying to look for cases that we thought might be COVID, and then sending the samples to Atlanta.

Initially, the turnaround was pretty quick, two to three days. But then you saw the surge occurring on the Mainland, first in Washington State, and the turnaround started to get slower and slower.

The State of Hawai'i Laboratories Division was the first state lab in any state to get certified to test for COVID. They were certified on February 28, and so we at least began to be able to test locally, which made a huge difference just in terms of the turnaround. We didn't have to compete with other states, and obviously the case counts in Hawai'i were really low compared to any place else. We knew that if we were not able to test locally we would go to the bottom of the pile—there definitely was a lot more virus activity in other states.

That made a tremendous difference. We knew that we had to be able to test in order to identify who was infected.

Kirk Caldwell So, Governor, at that meeting in Washington with the other governors, was there a sense of urgency, and did the topic of COVID occupy a large part of the conversation, or were most governors just becoming aware of it?

David Ige I do think that more than half the governors realized that it was a serious situation. It just depends on their state and whether they had experience with previous kinds of outbreaks. So it was interesting because the leaders in the federal government, the department heads, knew that it was serious, but because Trump didn't want the federal government to lead they made it clear that we should do everything we could to get test kits and personal protective equipment on our own.

When I went up to DC, the CDC had just prepared the test kits so that states could test, but the first batch of test kits they sent out was faulty. Our lab had run the tests and they didn't work.

I was trying to personally get kits in DC that I could take back because we knew that we had to test locally. I made a couple of calls, we were prepared to take corrected kits back, and then they said that the refabricated test kits had failed as well. They just were not ready.

Ron Mizutani, president of Hawai'i Foodbank, knew he could not wait for data to confirm that Hawai'i was heading for a food security crisis.

Ron Mizutani I was deeply concerned from the immediate word that this was happening in Asia. I actively started to do research on this virus and understood that this was coming our way no matter what we thought or said. I also watched how this was impacting the food banks in Asia and how it was impacting behaviors in Asia when it came to food and food insecurity. That was my job here at the time, so I knew it was going to affect us in a great way.

It would take a while to get to Hawai'i, but by January I was already informing our board and by February we were already making active purchases long before we even had our first positive case in the Islands. It was just kind of foresight, but also understanding what we were witnessing on television: empty shelves in Asia and people frantically purchasing products off shelves—stuff that we see often during hurricane season. That behavior is not new or unique to the Islands. I anticipated that this was definitely coming our way. When, I didn't know.

But I also knew that getting food here to the Islands, because we're so geographically isolated, takes time. And if this became an issue, where hoarding would start, the impact would be really great on food. Not just on Hawai'i Foodbank, but all nonprofits, all social services that provide food and shelter for those impacted by hunger. So, we actively made purchases that we had not budgeted for in anticipation of food shortfalls and especially food not being donated to Hawai'i Foodbank.

Once that first case was announced here in the Islands, I went directly to my media friends and said, "Hey look, we're not seeing it yet, but we will in the next few days. And I'd like to get ahead of it and plead to the public to not hoard and not do what we usually do when it came to crisis and when it came to disasters." I went on the air with three of my friends in the television world. All three stations, they actually came to the food bank, and I just shared my story of this virus. "It's here. We need to be mindful of each other and take care of each other. I understand protecting and taking care of your home and preparing your families for disaster, but if you can keep in mind those who have hunger as a crisis every day, this will affect Hawai'i Foodbank."

I'll be very honest with you. I got a lot of criticism from the community, some people actually cussing at me and saying, *How dare you tell us what to do! We're going to take care of our families if we need to.* The hoarding started shortly after. And that's when it had an impact on Hawai'i Foodbank in donations from the community. It just quickly became an issue. Thankfully, we did have some food on the way that carried us through the early months of the pandemic, but had we not had the foresight to make some of those preemptive purchases we would have been in a world of hurt.

Before the first case arrived, we actually even ordered N95 masks long before N95 was an acronym people knew and PPE (personal protection equipment) and all that stuff became part of our everyday lives. We were way ahead of the game so by the time people were starting to snatch up these masks, we already had distributed to our staff.

Ron Mizutani is a familiar name in the Islands. He worked as a television news reporter and anchor for decades and was also an executive of local utility Hawaiian Telcom. Ron's parents were born and raised on Kaua'i and his family knew firsthand how to survive in the aftermath of hurricanes and storms.

Ron Mizutani Some of it was my experience covering disasters and watching my family live through two hurricanes, Iwa and Iniki, knowing how quickly things, supplies, can be depleted. Some of it was just trusting my instinct. We were doing things that were so out of the box, and, frankly, it took some courage to make some of these decisions and, as I've said, some of that I got pushback from.

I trusted my instincts, trusted our team, and trusted the research that we did on our own. We just did things that were not part of our mission in some way. And that took a lot of guts and it also took a lot of failures. We definitely had some missteps along the way, but I look back on them and have no regrets. We did so many things right as opposed to doing things wrong.

Dr. Jonathan Dworkin is the author of the book The Plague Doctors, *about the role of doctors in Hawai'i during the first year of the pandemic. We first met him when he was invited to be part of the mayor's medical advisory group, which met every Thursday evening in the mayor's conference room, socially distanced, and also virtually. He quickly established himself as an invaluable resource to the administration. Specializing in internal medicine and infectious diseases at Queen's Medical Center, he started monitoring the virus long before it evolved into a global pandemic.*

Jonathan Dworkin There are infections that emerge continuously, so when you hear about a new infection emerging, as an ID (infectious diseases) person, you're not automatically alarmed by that because one of the big trends in infectious disease in the last few decades has been an increasing emergence of infections. And most of them end up being local problems; most of them don't become big, global pandemics. So, your default is not to assume that something is going to become a pandemic.

But there were some signs early on that got my attention, that alarmed me, and one of the things I found useful was around January or so, the World Health Organization (WHO) started putting out situation reports. And if you read those situation reports carefully what you saw was cases being reported country by country of the novel coronavirus.

I was not entirely trusting of the Chinese data. Not because they don't do good science; they do excellent science in China. But anything that touches on a political narrative in that country can become difficult to know what to do with in terms of your information. So I started charting the non-China cases. I actually had a little table on my computer and each day I would update it. This was late January, early February.

If you were doing that, what you saw was those countries with very good public health systems—places like Singapore, Japan—were having little clusters of cases. Not a large number, but it was obvious that the thing can spread beyond Wuhan and beyond the borders of China. Even places with excellent public health responses were having trouble controlling it. They would have zero cases for a few days and then *bam*, they had five cases. This kind of thing was going on. So you didn't have to see a massive outbreak outside China before you realized that this thing was leaking. The data was all there in the WHO reports going all the way back to January. You could have completely ignored the China data and still seen that happening.

And what happened was, as cases started to go up, that little trickle became dwarfed by the new case counts, and you couldn't see it on the graph anymore. But if you go back to the WHO situation reports, which I think are still posted, you can see even in January, early February, this trickle of cases. So that was the first thing that really got my attention. I thought, boy, they're not really containing this thing in Wuhan. And you don't have to trust the Chinese government, you don't have to trust any one government—you can triangulate between the reports coming out of different countries and see that they're having trouble containing this.

And then I thought, what would alarm me? In my mind, I roughly defined in advance what would alarm me, and that would be if we see a big jump in the non-China cases over a short period of time. So we go from one or two, and now we're at ten to twenty, and now we're at one hundred to two hundred, and we see a lot of rhythmic rise in the non-China cases over a short period of time—that means the thing hasn't just gone beyond the borders of China but is now exponentially growing. That would fulfill my criteria for "it's likely to go pandemic."

I was talking to some other very smart people at the time and we were trying to work through where the line was that we'd draw to say, okay, this is a big deal. Most of us agreed that that big steep rise in cases outside China would qualify.

I was talking to a guy named Masayuki Nogi who's a very bright general internist at Queen's, who comes from Japan and has academic connections in Japan, and we were looking at the Japanese data early on. That was where some of the earliest cases were reported, and they were the number two country at the very beginning, so we were thinking, okay, it's going to come to Hawai'i through Japanese air travel. We were wrong about that. But we were looking at those data every day together. This is like late January, early February.

And then the virus threw us a curveball, as it did so many times afterwards. The first big curveball it threw us was the big explosion in cases in Korea and Italy and Iran. So suddenly there's these three big clusters outside China and I don't know if you remember but those were the three countries that got hammered right after China. And they were all around the same time, within a week or two of each other. So at that point, that's around mid-February, I thought, okay, this thing is going to go pandemic.

Not only is it beyond China, but it's growing explosively in other countries. And that's when I stopped reassuring people. You have to understand, at the time, the American federal authorities were still kind of minimizing it. There were a lot of people going on TV saying, *Oh, the threat is low. The risk to the American population is low.* I stopped talking like that around mid-February; I thought that was irresponsible at that point. It was obviously exiting China and there was no way anybody was going to contain it. And that should have been the time, in my opinion, that the federal authorities in the United States should have started painting a darker picture and preparing people.

But we still had about a month of BS to go through before we got to the point where people were taking it very seriously. I often felt that I was the raving lunatic in the room towards the end of February. When you're the person saying, "Oh my god, something bad is coming our way," and 80 percent of the people around you don't agree, you feel kind of silly. People tell you you're panicking. You get this kind of feedback, which is negative essentially, like you're spreading anxiety for no good reason.

Peter Ingram is president and CEO of Hawaiian Airlines and its parent company, Hawaiian Holdings, Inc. He joined Hawaiian Airlines as chief financial officer in November 2005 and served as executive vice president and chief commercial officer from 2011 to 2018. We interviewed Peter in a small conference room adjacent to his "corner office," which is basically a humble cubicle space within a large bullpen of other staff cubicles. He's tall and lanky, and it's no surprise that his last trip before the world locked down combined a business conference with a Duke–North Carolina basketball game before he headed home to Hawaiʻi.

Peter Ingram For us, it started in February. It began as an impact on demand for some of our Asia flights. First, South Korea, and then Japan. So as the virus had jumped more significantly from China to Korea, we started to see traffic falling off. We had a global sales meeting sometime in mid-February with all of our sales people from around the world and as we were watching demand deteriorate rapidly on our Korea flights, we realized there would be a severe impact on our business and on Hawaiʻi.

At that time, we were thinking the effect might be significant on only a portion of our network, not our complete network. Our context for thinking about it at the time was something more like SARS or bird flu or MERS, which were all regional. We weren't in a mindset, at that point, of thinking about a global pandemic.

That impact on bookings and cancellations then went to Japan. Then we started to see it on some of our domestic flights. Now we're probably into the early part of March. By late February we suspended our Korea service. We started reducing our Japan schedule, so we took some frequencies out of our multifrequency markets like Tokyo and we suspended our Sapporo flight in early March.

In the first week in March, we had an Airlines for America (A4A) board meeting. A4A is our national trade association, and we had a regular quarterly meeting in Washington, DC. Not only was everyone talking about COVID, we had a meeting scheduled to go and meet Vice President Mike Pence to discuss the severe impact this was going to have on the airline industry, again thinking largely internationally, but starting to spill into domestic. I don't think any of us knew the magnitude of what was to come. We actually went to the White House and we not only met with Pence but President Trump joined the meeting also. There was no CARES Act under discussion at that point and we were explicitly not asking for anything except for the government to support us in terms of policy.

The world changed pretty quickly. I went to visit my daughter and attend the Duke–North Carolina basketball game on the way home at the end of that week, which was the last fun thing I did before the world changed dramatically. For the rest of March, we were constantly changing our schedule because we would publish a new schedule to reflect cancellations and reduction in demand. And then before we could even get that out, things had gotten worse. Australia and New Zealand put entry restrictions in place, so we canceled our flights to Australia and New Zealand. The domestic cases started to mount, and I can't remember when we started seeing it on our New York route, but we were pulling our schedule down long before the Hawai'i quarantine.

Before being appointed as director of the DOH (Hawai'i State Department of Health) in September 2020, Dr. Elizabeth "Libby" Char began monitoring the virus while working at the City and County of Honolulu as the medical director for the Honolulu Fire Department. She is an emergency medicine physician.

Libby Char In January, we heard about the problem in China. And I think most people here, me as well, were thinking it was going to be like SARS or MERS-CoV or one of those other diseases; that it stays there, somewhere on the Mainland, or international, but doesn't make its way here.

And then in February we started seeing the numbers go up, and as soon as we saw the cases in Seattle, we started getting worried. I started getting worried. If it's in Seattle, what's to prevent it from coming here? It's a plane ride away. That's when I started becoming concerned, but was still hoping it would be something that would, like MERS-CoV, kind of peter out.

At the time, we didn't know enough about the characteristics of it to know if it would in fact do what a few bad infectious diseases had done. We were cautiously watching.

I was talking with the state epidemiologist at the time, and because I wasn't really looped in with the state system beyond that, I was mostly talking to my colleagues on the Mainland. There's a group of metropolitan medical directors for EMS and a lot of really smart people in that group including guys that are double boarded in infectious diseases and a lot of research folks. So I had mostly been talking to them to hear what was going on in other states, what they were seeing, and what they thought in terms of if this was going to be something that was going to blow up in the United States or not.

Seattle has a really strong public health department. Those guys factored prominently into sharing the information on what was known. An epidemiologist from CIDRAP (Center for Infectious Disease Research and Policy), Mike Osterholm, was on many of those calls. It was really valuable to have firsthand conversations with someone like him because he had a good global perspective and a ton of experience. And when we started hearing Seattle get really nervous about it and all of a sudden their numbers, particularly in their care homes, started to go up and their first responders were getting sick, that's when the realization really hit that we'd better do something.

Also in this group are medical directors from London, Germany, Italy, Ireland, France, Australia, so we had a pretty good representation on what was going on globally as well as just in the United States.

The UK and Italy were having huge issues. People were dying in Italy. Seattle cases started increasing and once New York began experiencing tremendous disease burden, I think that's when everybody really just hit the brakes.

From a City standpoint, as far back as early February we were having those discussions internally with EMS and the Honolulu Fire Department (HFD) because the firefighters were wanting to know when they responded to calls if they need to do anything differently, what kind of PPE to use, and all of that. We really were paying attention to the safety measures. The City started having briefings, but I wasn't initially invited to those. I kind of snuck into some of them anyway and there were some firefighters there, so I would talk to them right after the meeting and try and ask them for a recap. Then I just kind of started attending. I spoke with Hiro Toiya (director of DEM) and he was okay with me sitting in on the briefings. So I started sitting in a little bit more regularly. That was good to be able to get the daily updates and hear what was going on.

We had been having conversations internally in the fire department because knowing what was going on in Seattle, we were already trying to procure the PPE. We weren't sure if the federal government was going to do it or not, so we were kind of waiting for that, but by then we were checking our inventory. What do we have? How much? What's appropriate? What should we be wearing when we respond to 911 calls? How do we protect the firefighters and paramedics? Because at that point it became obvious that it would be a matter of when we get a case, not if.

Back in February, we knew there was a problem and I was working with Honolulu Fire, Maui Fire, Kauai Fire, AMR (American Medical Response) statewide, and conversing with the emergency physicians in the communities. We were concerned about it. And it highlighted one of the significant things in Hawaiʻi, which is similar to the DOE (Hawaiʻi State Department of Education) and to EMS. We have a statewide health department, but we have no county public health department.

Obviously, there's good and bad in that, because the DOH usually is focused on regulatory and administrative and guidance, and not as much on a large response at the operational level. And that was really significant because there was an expectation by the public that the DOH would do something. And yet the DOH doesn't necessarily have the structure or the number of people sufficient to act as responders to actually implement *all* of the guidelines and the guidance. So that was a bit of a disconnect. There was an expectation by the State that the Counties would help to do that. And yet the expectation by the Counties was that that was a State *kuleana*. And I think that was problematic for Hawaiʻi because there was a gap there and no one really had ownership of that gap. By and large, some of the County response agencies had to step in beyond what they normally do to try to fill some of that gap.

In the long run it worked out well because I think in Hawaiʻi we have much more of a sense of community. But from an administrative standpoint, it was a little bit rough in the beginning. It didn't seem like there was top-down clarity on who was responsible for what. By default, the Counties sort of stepped up and the State stretched beyond their usual daily activities.

Micah Kane is CEO and president of the Hawaiʻi Community Foundation (HCF). As we started interviewing the leaders for this book, it quickly became apparent that a trifecta had formed early on between

Peter Ho, Ray Vara, and Micah Kane. They were looking at data, becoming concerned with what they were seeing, and anticipating the worst if nothing was done. As Ho said, when they talked to others, it was a little like "barking at the moon."

Micah Kane Late February, there was already an ad hoc group of people that were communicating, via group text, organically. And Ray Vara was a big piece of that information pool because you needed someone who was thinking from a medical standpoint, and the implications from the health standpoint, and he was the first one to start forecasting what the implications would be if it did come here without any of the restrictions that you, Mayor, contemplated. He was already saying, okay, if we do this, this is how we can flatten the curve; if we do this, this is how we can further flatten the curve; here's the sensitivity that these conditions have to our economic well-being. Here's the correlation between those restrictions and our economy. And then we were laying out a framework. Regardless of what framework you adopt, you need something that is going to allow you to communicate to the public how you're going to be making decisions. It's going to be imperfect, but you need something.

Peter Ho (Bank of Hawai'i) By now, it's into February. And it's very interesting because, clearly, we thought this was a State issue, and if you go back to that period, the posture was that, boy, it would be really inconvenient to slow things down around here. And not too different from any place else in the country. First of all, there's no precedence, so how would you know? And second of all, no one's really making a big deal about it, so why should we make a big deal about it? So we were kind of like barking at the moon. But it was really me, Ray, and Micah. We were pretty aligned. We just felt Hawai'i had the opportunity to be effective in thwarting the virus. So why not try?

And the other thing that's interesting is that I remember reading an analysis that one of the big accounting firms had put out—this is going back years—an analysis of places in the world where global pandemics would be especially devastating. And Hawai'i was one of them. And the reason why it was one of them was because we really over-indexed in terms of air travel relative to the size of the population, because of what we do for a living. But if you reverse that, kind of the opposite becomes true. You can inoculate yourself from the rest of the world.

Before government took any action on travel quarantines or lockdowns, some private companies saw the writing on the wall early on and decided to go ahead and implement safety measures in the workplace. They got ahead of the curve, and one of them was Alexander & Baldwin. Chris Benjamin is the president and CEO of this premier commercial real estate company, which has managed business, retail, and industrial properties in Hawai'i for over 150 years.

Chris Benjamin I don't remember when I first heard about COVID-19, but I remember when I first got worried about it. I flew through Houston to Orlando on February 25, 2020. And by the time I landed in Orlando and got to my hotel, a number of things had triggered in me the realization that this was coming and this was going to be bad and we had to do something about it.

I was on my way to a conference, and I don't even remember what data points I was collecting, but I think I was reading the paper, I was seeing CNN, I was seeing some early precautions being put into place. No one was wearing masks, of course. The big thing at that point was all about washing your hands. It wasn't so much about the airborne aspects of the virus.

I remember that at this conference I attended, it was the first time I'd ever seen a men's room where the guys were standing in line to wash their hands because people were following the twenty-second hand washing guidance.

But the day that I landed in Orlando, I got to my hotel and called Lance Parker (executive vice president and chief real estate officer) and I said, "We've got to stand up a task force. We've got to get ahead of this. Because this is coming." And I think I would have been surprised at that point if you had told me that two weeks later our office would be shut down.

By the time I got back on March 4, we had had several meetings, and by the following Wednesday—I think it was March 11—we had sent everybody home.

We did it early. Here's why. When you know something's inevitable, why take chances? The most important thing facilitating our being very early on was the fact that everybody in the company had a laptop, everybody had remote file storage, and everybody had access to Teams. This task force included our IT executives and we figured out very early on that we could do remote meetings and we could do all this stuff virtually, so I just decided, well, why not? So, March 11, we sent people home. If they needed to be in the office on March 12 and 13—I think that was the Thursday and Friday—they could come in, but by the end of Friday it had to be virtual.

The following Monday, I think the banks followed. It was pretty quick. From my perspective, I don't think we had many slow adopters in Hawai'i. I think people were pretty conscientious about it.

It's funny because you look back at some of the decisions that you thought were bold and progressive at the time, and three days later they seem so obvious. Like how could you have ever thought you wouldn't do that? But it was over a matter of days things went from being not so obvious to being very obvious.

At the end of February, Dr. Jonathan Dworkin's clarion call on the impending pandemic was getting him into some hot water. He posted his position on Facebook and the reaction from the community was swift.

Jonathan Dworkin (Queen's Health System) Initially, it was a lot of conversations. The first of the Facebook posts that got me in trouble, I published on February 29, a leap day, and I said it was going to go pandemic. I thought about that post a lot before I put it up because I realized I was throwing a grenade. I think I edited it two or three times. Usually, I'm posting pictures of my kids and stuff; I'm not that thoughtful. But that one I took seriously, and I wrote a very careful post and I put it out there. I got about a hundred comments, it got shared a hundred times, people were emailing me afterwards. A lot of people were saying, "Hey, all we've been hearing is this kind of false reassurance narrative. This is the first time someone we know has really raised a red flag." So I got a lot of positive feedback on that. And people thanked me for sort of clarifying what was coming our way.

JONATHAN DWORKIN'S FEBRUARY 29, 2020 FACEBOOK POST

Coronavirus: Is it overhyped?

There seems to be a lot of confusion about this, so it's a topic worthy of a deeper look.

When confronted with a new problem, most people have a bias towards their initial reaction. We look for data points that confirm our view and reassure us that we are reading the situation correctly. We also tend to be biased towards the status quo.

What was my initial bias towards coronavirus? That it was being overhyped. In infectious diseases, the discovery of new infections is increasingly common, both because our population has grown and become more global and because we have increasingly powerful tools to detect and describe new pathogens.

That means it's hard for me to get too excited by a new bug. When Ebola re-emerged a few years ago, I was interested but honestly didn't spend too much time on it. I had actual patients with other infections to worry about and I judged (correctly) that the risk to the United States was low. And those powerful new tools also reassured me. We had this novel coronavirus sequenced almost as soon as it was detected. Vaccine development is happening at a pace that was unimaginable when I was a child.

But as I paid more attention to the new virus, my hot take began to chill. I want to explain why and what data points I am looking at. It's not going to be possible to get everyone to agree on what the actual threat level is, but the less confused we are about the parameters, the more useful the discourse.

The first thing that worried me was the data on transmission outside China. The situation in China is bad, but interpreting what's going on there is hard (at least for me) because of the chaotic nature of their situation: case definitions have changed more than once, resources in Wuhan were stretched to the breaking point, and the government has a media narrative (a.k.a. propaganda) that it is pushing.

So, in order to unconfuse myself, I ignored the China data and began reading the part of the daily WHO report that deals with non-China infections. And if you read those reports, you see that even weeks ago there was community transmission occurring in neighboring countries. Not much. A few cases here and there in places like Singapore, Malaysia, and Japan. That trickle of cases was alarming because it indicated that containment measures were not succeeding.

Next, I defined for myself what would indicate a serious threat. The parameter I came up with was a logarithmic increase in non-China cases, particularly if that occurred over a relatively short time scale (i.e., a couple weeks, the expected latency period of the virus). When the Korean outbreak began in earnest in late February and we started seeing additional clusters in Italy and Iran, that criteria was fulfilled.

That's when I stopped reassuring people. And that's when I found myself becoming frustrated by confused comparisons of the new virus with other infections, many of which (failing to account for the high rate of transmission) were intended to downplay its significance. I think the people speaking this way—some of them doctors—were well-intentioned. But I also think they weren't paying attention.

If you look at the measures being taken in countries heavily impacted by the new virus in order to control it, what you see is a level of disruption that few people alive are accustomed to: prolonged closures of public spaces, quarantines of entire towns, a massive decrease in air travel and public transit. What this amounts to is a major disruption in cultural and economic activity. And those measures seem to be slowing, but not stopping, the spread of the virus.

It's not the apocalypse, but it's not normal life either.

So, my level of worry is correspondingly high, and I think the data supports that.

Now that said, in order to keep myself honest, I should define once again what would change my mind. What needs to happen to convince me that this is being overhyped?

I can think of two big data points that are worth tracking. One is the fatality rate of the infection. If we find out that there's a massive number of barely symptomatic cases we are missing, and the true fatality rate is much lower than has been reported (i.e., 0.1%, as opposed to 2%), that would be reassuring. That would be mortality that's actually more on par with a flu season. A bad deal, but not as alarming as the current numbers suggest. (And I should point out that we don't yet have good data on mild or asymptomatic illness, so I expect some revision down in the fatality rate.) This scenario is possible, though a pandemic of a new virus with flu-like mortality would still be a big deal.

The other reassuring data point would be a decrease in transmission. Ebola was highly fatal, but I didn't worry much about it because the likelihood it would spread far without detection was low. If I see a similar pattern with coronavirus (i.e., containment is successful and the non-China cases begin to drop), that too will be soothing. But on this front, the minimally symptomatic cases actually work against us (and may well be why containment has been failing).

Right now I am not seeing either of those data points shift dramatically, which is why I think the only responsible advice to give people is to prepare themselves for a significant disruption in ordinary life. A pandemic with a mortality of even 1% would be a very big deal. Which means that vacation you want to take is not as important as making sure you don't become a vector for someone's aging mother. Telehealth and tele-education should boom right now. Netflix should do a brisk business. And helping each other through an emergency is more important than pursuing our usual pleasures and ambitions.

Jonathan Dworkin So there was that which I did in public. In private, there were a lot of interactions with the Queen's administration that I was having at that time trying to get them prepared. One of the questions that you sent me, Mayor, was about regrets. The year before, I had the opportunity to be the infectious disease chief at Queen's and

I turned it down. As a young doctor I thought, well, someday I'll be the chief of infectious disease and that will be great, a little feather in my cap, as a career person. And then I get to be kind of middle-aged with family and we're coming over to Waimea and I have more patients here on the Big Island and we're thinking about moving my practice over and I'm trying to spend more time with my wife and kids, and I thought, I don't want to go to all these meetings. What is this job going to give me that's really going to improve my life? Am I really going to be able to make that big of an impact? Probably not. So I said no.

This is just a few months before the pandemic. And then the pandemic's coming and I'm thinking, *Boy, wouldn't it be nice to be the infectious disease chief right now? I could really focus the conversation for the whole state from that perch.* But I excluded myself from that role.

Now, I'm knocking on the door very politely and saying, "Guys, I know I'm not the chief, I just said no, but this is really a big problem. Can we talk? Can we at least let me in the room so we can have these conversations?" And to their credit—it's a very professional place—I was still welcomed in almost every important conversation, and in the end, it wasn't that big a deal. People who ran the division did an excellent job, I think.

A lot of the people, including some very smart people, had tremendous faith in the CDC and the DOH. Essentially, what I was saying was I don't think they're getting it right. I think we need to develop a lab-developed test. I was saying stuff like, "Don't even wait for FDA approval. Break the law and get us a test so we can start testing people." So you can imagine how that advice went over in a place that usually follows every single rule to a T, because they're required to. And I'm saying, "Let them sue you. Let them come arrest us. It's better if we have a test that we can use in an emergency room, and they can explain why they're arresting us for testing people. Let's just have the test."

It was tense. I would say it was very tense. But one of the things that was interesting was how quickly the thinking changed. So in a matter of a couple of weeks we went from "don't stir up panic" and "we don't need to test anybody" to "we're going to test every single admission that comes into the hospital," once we actually had the approval to do the test.

And it went from "we don't need to wear masks at all" to "everybody who walks in the building or near the building has got to wear a mask and get a temperature screen regardless." I think the testing became available in the middle of March. The universal masking, for outside the hospital, was a little later—I want to say April. But in the hospital, it started a little earlier and we essentially did like what we call universal flu precautions. So that's like when there's a bad flu season, we just make everybody mask so that we don't have transmission of fluid in the hospital. And that was something I pushed early on: *Why don't we just start doing that now?* There were issues with supplies as well, but eventually that's what they did. We've been doing universal flu precautions ever since.

But early on it was not evident that everybody needed to do those types of things. And the testing in particular would create a tension because we had the CDC saying we don't need to test unless someone has a specific travel history to Wuhan. And then they expanded it; not just Wuhan but Korea or Italy. And I'm looking at these WHO situation reports, saying, "Guys, it's not just in those places. It's already spread all over the place. It might already be on the continent. These geographic testing requirements don't make sense anymore." So, I'm sending out increasingly desperate emails.

Over time, what I was saying looked more true. And the testing resource became more available. And then we started doing more universal testing and it was really private testing that I think saved us. DLS (Diagnostic Laboratory Services) developed a test that became available through the Queen's system. And that was like the lights turning on. Up until then we were operating in the dark. Suddenly, we had a floodlight and we could see exactly where the virus was.

Scott Miskovich did something similar with community testing and Clinical Labs, and got a lot of scorn heaped on him by the DOH for doing that. He was one hundred percent right and did a lot of good by doing that. These things were the kinds of arguments that were happening early on. I kind of nudged my way back into the conversation at Queen's. Eventually, they set up a clinical trials group that they invited me to be on where a lot of COVID issues got discussed. And of course, I was on the COVID call schedule because I was still in the Division of

Infectious Diseases, so I was seeing the patients.

As for everyone else, there was an adjustment, but we did adjust.

As the head of Hawai'i Pacific Health, Ray Vara is responsible for the oversight of Straub Medical Center, Kapi'olani Medical Center, Pali Momi Medical Center, and Wilcox Medical Center on Kaua'i. HPH's annual board retreat is an important event for the organization. It went forward successfully, but on the same day Hawai'i saw its first case of COVID-19.

Ray Vara Our annual board retreat started on March 6, 2020. This includes all of our board members, physician leaders, spouses, and executive management. It's something that we plan for all year. We bring in a world-class speaker who can share a message consistent with the key strategies we are rolling out. That year our speaker was Wes Moore, the CEO of the Robin Hood Foundation in New York.

March 6 was also the day the first COVID case arrived in Hawai'i. As you can imagine, in the weeks leading up to our retreat, as cases rose around the country, the question was whether we do the retreat or not. So, on Thursday, March 5, I made the decision that we're going to do it. There were no cases yet in Hawai'i and we had all the protective measures in place: hand sanitizers available, a plan for social distancing, no hugging, no shaking hands. That said, we certainly weren't sitting six feet apart. Had we known then what we know now, we would never have done that event. It was the last big event in Honolulu, and it could have been disastrous. I guess sometimes it is better to be lucky rather than good.

Shortly thereafter, we stood up our command centers across the system, which centralized all of our leadership. We have a command center structure much like the State and City and County Emergency Operations Center (EOC).

Derek Kawakami is the mayor of Kaua'i County, which includes the islands of Kaua'i and Ni'ihau. The first reported case of COVID on Kaua'i was on March 13, 2020. His managing director, Mike Dahilig, became concerned about a possible pandemic as early as January.

Derek Kawakami Fortunately, Mike was aware of it as he had watched it grow from this respiratory illness in China. Then he went to a "disaster camp." I think the camp was started some time ago by [former Hawai'i US senator] Daniel Inouye, but it's all based around FEMA and disaster management. But they were on the Big Island and they had a speaker talk to them and every day on his breaks Mike would call us.

The only real thing that sunk in for me was on March 13, at about 9:30 or 10:00 at night, when I got the call that we had our first confirmed case. And I knew it was going to be an issue. I don't think I fully realized how big an issue it was going to be, but I do remember when we had our first confirmed positives who were visitors. That's when it sunk in. And I'm not one to get rattled, but I gotta say that I came into the EOC that evening with a cold sweat. I knew that we were going to get some cases.

Our guys had gotten furniture and they were just starting to furnish our isolation center. And I remember calling our unified commander, Sol Kanoho, and I asked him, "What's the status of you folks wrapping this up tonight?" He said, "We're going to come back tomorrow and finish it." I said, "No, you guys are gonna finish this up, because we're going to move our two positives from the hotel to the isolation center." I was met with resistance all around. They were not happy campers.

Our district health officer and her counterparts were concerned that the hotel had said, "They can stay overnight. They're safe. We'll get them out there tomorrow." I said, "We're getting them out of there tonight." I just told them, "Look, I'm gonna make a call. I'll tell you what's going to happen: the hotel workers are going to find out that we have the first two positive cases in the hotel; our office is going to be flooded with angry husbands, kids, and wives asking us why we didn't inform anybody." So, we moved them out. They were healthy enough to be transported out to our isolation center and the next morning my district health officer said, "You made the right call." At the end of the day, I'm the only one that's going to be held accountable for this thing. If it fails, I will accept it. And if we succeed, we succeed as a team.

Sure enough, the couple had called room service and told the staff, "By the way, we're COVID positive." And I said, "These things happen.

It's called the coconut wireless. And this is why we gotta move." That was the first real definitive time where I said, "You guys may all have opinions, and I take them all to heart, but at the end of the day my call is my call. And that's it. There's one button and one person that's going to get to push that button. You guys just follow me, and we'll get through this."

Leadership can be a very lonely position, and we asked how he managed that.

Derek Kawakami I've always been okay being alone. That's one thing. My wife thinks it's pretty interesting that when I travel for work I have no problem going to a restaurant just eating by myself. I grew up pretty much as a latchkey kid. My brothers were way older than me. When we moved to Kaua'i, they were at boarding schools, Kamehameha and Mid-Pacific. My dad was busy running a business, and my mom was busy as a schoolteacher. And even when I was on O'ahu in kindergarten and first grade, I had to learn how to take the public transportation to get from Mililani Uka back home. And I also rode around to get to where my mom taught or to Pearlridge. My mom grew up very poor and my dad grew up in a family that was scratching and clawing to be successful, and so I think they knew they had to teach their kids how to survive. I think that, in a sense, helps me out because you know, and I know, that it is lonely but I'm quite okay being lonely.

Throughout the course of the pandemic, we admired the professionalism and sound medical recommendations coming from Kaua'i's district health officer, Dr. Janet Berreman.

Derek Kawakami Absolutely. Dr. Berreman, she was the district health officer at Berkeley when H1N1 came through, so she's had some experience with it, but no matter what, I'm always going to turn to the most knowledgeable subject matter expert in the room. If it's a fire, I'm not going to turn to the district health officer. That's where I think I saw things fall apart—from the very top, when they made this pandemic a political issue. So what was happening was the voices from the health community and medical community, their voices were being muffled. And they were being thrown in what I'd say is the misinformation stew, which really created confusion. Which to me was the bigger problem than the virus itself. At a time when we needed a leader to bring our country together, they were still very much focused on creating a divide. I think that's a lesson to be learned no matter what party you're in, no matter if you're a politician or not. You could just be a regular average joe and realize that if you take the route of fear and guilt to create a division, it's a very powerful tool, but it's the least effective way of solving problems. And I hope that future leaders choose the path of being clear, having confidence, bringing people together, because once you go down the road of fear, guilt and confusion, and divisiveness it's hard to roll that back and bring the people back together again. It's hard to build trust. Only time will heal that wound.

Harry Kim is the former mayor of Hawai'i County, which is often referred to as the Big Island of Hawai'i. He has been a public figure on the Big Island since the 1970s, primarily as the civil defense director for twenty-four years. He's no stranger to crisis management, and his name is synonymous with natural disasters, from active volcanoes and earthquakes to tsunamis.

Harry Kim I was in civil defense for twenty-four years. I went into that department not knowing anything. It was after the island of Hawai'i experienced a 7.5 earthquake in 1975, which caused a local tsunami, destruction, and unfortunately fatalities. Not knowing much about the job, I called people all over the world to learn from their experiences. A very important thing to know was that the responsibilities and functions of civil defense at that time for the United States was literally still in its infancy. Still, a lot of the emphasis on training was focused on preparation for war. Also, the knowledge and responses for natural disasters were still in the learning stages. One of the most important things I learned was our failure in responses for disasters. I concluded that the very basic reason for failure was compounded because of the lack of trust in government during emergencies. Due to that, I established as a major goal to work towards the trust of government.

Harry Kim is a voracious reader and consumer of news. As he tracked what was happening around the world, he became the first mayor to put out a civil defense message on pandemic planning, dated Tuesday, February 4, 2020.

This is an information update on the coronavirus for Tuesday, February 4, 2020, at noon. A partnership was formed—key agencies from federal, state, and county government, along with the medical community—to assure you receive timely and accurate information about the virus. This partnership is committed to providing the residents of Hawai'i County the most reliable and accurate information available. As part of this partnership, an informational pamphlet is now being developed that addresses the most frequently asked questions, which will be ready for distribution this Friday—information provided by Civil Defense on what you need to know about the virus, health advisories, and actions taken by government. Daily updates on issues that may affect you and the coronavirus will be provided by Civil Defense. For more information call Civil Defense at 935-0031, Department of Health at 974-6001, Department of Health after hours at 211. This is your Hawai'i County Civil Defense.

Mayor Kim declared a state of emergency on February 28, 2020. At that time, there were zero cases of coronavirus reported in Hawai'i. He visited Governor David Ige, the Hawai'i Emergency Management Agency (HI-EMA), and the DOH and urged them to set up a central command, keeping in mind that he had already sounded the alarm publicly on February 4.

He remembers his reading on the nature of pandemics.

Harry Kim Coronavirus is a pandemic that can be worldwide and there are several very important issues about all pandemics that we must know. One, it is new, meaning we know very little about it. Because of its newness, we're going to learn as we go and we're going to have to change as we go. To do this, government must establish a system to monitor it to enable us to make timely changes as necessary.

Dennis Francis is the president and publisher of Oahu Publications, which includes MidWeek, various specialty publications, and the largest daily newspaper in Hawai'i, the Honolulu Star-Advertiser. *As the pandemic started to exponentially spread beyond China, the news coverage became even more important as a source of reliable information.*

Dennis Francis The editors understood the huge significance of this story and it quickly became our top story every day for many months. I think we did an excellent job of localizing the story so that the community understood what was happening in Hawai'i. Of course, we devoted space to the national and world pandemic news, but our number one job was reporting on the local impact. The pandemic affected every aspect of life in Hawai'i, and our staff worked incredibly hard to explain it all and to share what resources were available to help people cope.

Christina Kishimoto was the superintendent of the DOE from 2017 to the end of her contract in July 2021. It's hard to imagine a tougher job than managing a statewide public school system during a health crisis and balancing the needs of children, support for teachers, mental and physical health, safety, food insecurity, cooperation of parents, and the lack of adequate resources for information technology that was required for distance learning.

Christina Kishimoto In March, we were heading toward spring break and all of a sudden I was getting lots of questions: "Are you going to shut down?" And I thought, *Why am I going to shut down?*

Other jurisdictions were being asked the same question and were trying to figure this out. And then all of a sudden it was upon us and spring break was about to start, and we said, "Okay, we're going to extend spring break by one week to see what this is about." Two weeks later, we're saying, "I think we're shutting down for longer than two weeks." It was the regular spring break and we added a week for precaution, and then all hell broke loose.

Kishimoto had gone to Governor Ige to get his approval and agreement to not come back after spring break, essentially shutting down schools. The governor agreed with her but wanted to first have a discussion with the four mayors to get their consensus.

Christina Kishimoto I was thinking, *I don't think we can come back*, but there was so much confusion nationally. There was no consistency, no one really knew how to understand this, and so when I got together with the mayors all I was asking for was agreement with my decisions since the governor said he would agree, just so we have consistency of the decision makers—not that any of us knew what we were doing yet.

This was hard to understand. And what in the world? Now we're talking about masking and shutting down, and what does this all mean?

I am a board member of CCSSO (Council of Chief State School Officers). All fifty superintendents serve on that, as well as Guam, Puerto Rico, and US Virgin Islands. And also, the Department of Defense. So, there's fifty-four of us represented on that board. I'm on the executive board, which started having meetings almost every third day to check in on what in the world was going on, who's doing what, and that was an important team for me. So I would come back and meet with the governor and say, "This is the national conversation right now around who's doing what. This is not just about one neighborhood involved in a mudslide or a hurricane that is going to go by. This is a scary and little understood health pandemic. Let's just err on the side of precaution."

The worst-case scenario, I thought, was we're going to extend the school year. Everyone would be mad at me about extending the school year into the summer to make up lost instructional time, but that's not the worst thing that could happen. So I think it was just a matter of looking at what the options were, and the worst option was staying open and having kids and families get ill.

I drafted something for the governor and said, "I'm ready to send this out. I'm shutting down. What do you think?" Only because there was no time. So I said, "Here's the language. Can I work with your communications person? What do you think?" He said, "Okay, you're the leader and I'm going to back you." And I appreciate that he did that because I could have been wrong in my decision, but at the same time, as a leader, you know at the end of the day you've gotta make decisions. You can't just be spinning your wheels having everyone waiting for you to make a decision.

Just the whole idea of shutting down education—you're still accountable for it, so what do you do? And we've got teachers and principals quickly putting together paper packets because, again, we didn't even know how many electronic devices we had out there because we were not managing in that way. And so life changed very quickly on how to operationalize public education in a physical school shutdown.

UNUSUAL PARTNERSHIPS

In late February and early March, collaborations were forming within the community. Normally, collaborations form around groups with common interests, be it business, travel, nonprofits, government, health, data and research, etc. But the collaborations established during the pandemic were unique in that they brought together representatives from different groups with the understanding that COVID needed to be fought on many different fronts, tackled swiftly, in a race to survive the virus and its wake.

Mark Mugiishi describes himself as an optimist, and we would also add renaissance man. He is president and CEO of the Hawaii Medical Service Association (HMSA), the state's largest health insurance provider. He is a medical doctor and for most of his career had a private practice in general surgery and co-founded the Endoscopy Institute of Hawaii and the Eye Surgery Center of Hawaii. He has taught surgery at the John A. Burns School of Medicine and also currently serves as chair of the ʻIolani School Board of Governors. Perhaps he is best known in the community as varsity basketball coach for ʻIolani, leading the team to eleven league championships and seven state championships. What people might not know is that he was also the producer of the Broadway musical Allegiance starring George Takei and Lea Salonga, which ran at the Shubert's Longacre Theatre in New York City 2015–16.

Given HMSA's prominence in the medical community, Mark and his team were major players in one of the collaborations that helped lead the state through the pandemic.

Mark Mugiishi When it first started happening in other places around the world, my first reaction was we live on an island and it's very minimally going to come here. We're protected by the Pacific Ocean; I think we'll be fine. I think at one point China was number one and number two was a ship, the *Diamond Princess.* So it's not really going to be a big deal. When it started hitting other countries, then you start getting worried. Then when we had our first case, which was a tourist, then you go, *Okay, so it can breach our shores.*

I really became concerned for our state and our island around March when I started seeing that hospital capacity was being impacted.

I have frequent conversations with Queen's and HPH, and the people who run those hospitals, and they started saying things like, "Our ICUs are getting full." Then you get worried. Right around that time is when all of us shared with the governor that it was time to take stronger action because we're starting to get to a point of healthcare capacity issues.

In the beginning, obviously we didn't know a lot about this virus. Nobody knows the rate of transmission, what the characteristics are, how easily it infects people—all those things were big questions. So there was no book that says this is the way you address COVID and there was no data to say for sure if you looked at the data this is what you should do. So in the beginning, it was mainly scouring the globe for best practices.

You look at places that had issues before us; China was one, and then places with similar coronavirus type pandemics in the past—like Taiwan, Singapore, Japan—that had addressed those pretty well, whether it was SARS, MERS, or other things like that. What did they do to control those outbreaks? And you try and get best practices from them.

We looked at New Zealand because they're similar to us in that they're an island—they can control their borders. They were doing pretty well in the beginning, in spite of getting their first infections pretty early. They got on it right away and they controlled it, so we tried to follow some of their best practices.

And then we looked at big consulting groups with big staffs, like Boston Consulting Group and others, that could help us scour the world. So besides using all of the resources we had at our organization, we said go bigger, find as many people as possible in the world that are experienced at this kind of thing, and pick and choose from the best practices.

Blue Cross and Blue Shield Association has thirty-five member plans—thirty-six if you count Puerto Rico—across the US, and we have board meetings every other month. During COVID we just escalated that—we had them more often. And just sharing best practices, coming up with standard nationwide practices, testing practices, coverage practices, the best way to handle outbreaks—all those kinds of things. We did all those things, again, to try and share best practices.

Now, admittedly, healthcare is local, so you can have these kinds of blanket things but everyone's going to act a little differently in their own locale. It's also based on the way their own local governments act. For example, you're not going to have the same healthcare policies in Hawai'i, which were very protective in a "let's lock everything down and not let people out" kind of way, as you are going to have in Miami. Or basically places where it was "Do whatever you want. If you want a big gathering, go for it, and if people get sick, oh well. That's up to you, right?" So you have different kinds of approaches to that depending on the policy in your area.

One thing that was really good early on was that we were involved in this public-private partnership where we had a lot of public officials that included all the mayors and many private organizations like ourselves, HPH, Queen's, all that, and we tried to come up with a plan. Some kind of plan that would work for Hawai'i. This was our COVID-19 public-private task force. Just the fact that both elected officials and heads of private organizations got together and tried their best to create this plan gave our board, as well as, I think, the community, confidence that somebody was trying to collect the best information and come up with a plan. We came up with our own tier system and our own plan of action, including the pillars of screening, testing, and contact tracing, quarantine, all of those things, and the challenges that were with our

DOH in getting them operationalized. But the public-private partnership was the way to go because it helped start to build a cohesive plan and public confidence.

Who were the founding fathers and mothers of that plan?

Mark Mugiishi On the private side, mainly the healthcare organizations. So it was Ray Vara with HPH, Jill Hoggard Green with Queen's, myself with HMSA. Some of the banks; the big employers like Bob Harrison from First Hawaiian, Peter Ho from Bank of Hawaiʻi. The community foundations like Micah Kane was there. Public side: Speaker of the House, Senate president, the administration, the governor and his team, and county mayors were the people that we tried to bring in. We tried very hard to engage the DOH. Early on, it was a challenge to collaborate with them and they seemed to struggle to want to be part of it. Perhaps they figured they had it under control and they didn't need help. You know, a sort of "we got this" kind of mentality. Honestly that was the wrong mentality to have with something as serious as COVID sweeping across the world. This was a statewide, community-wide pandemic. A generational pandemic. Everybody had to be all hands on deck.

Another group also centered around business groups, banks, and data collection, including the Hawaiʻi Community Foundation (HCF) and the Hawaiʻi Executive Collaborative (HEC).

Micah Kane The Collaborative provided the ability to have broader reach into the leadership of our community faster. That's what Duane Kurisu has delivered—a network of leaders who are willing to look at our community through a common lens. Even at that level, it's around common data, shared goals, collective action. So if you're looking at the same set of data, imperfect data, at least it's benchmarked, place based. It's the best we got—let's agree that this is the data we're going to be making decisions from. From there, let's create some shared goals. Now let's have some collective action. Otherwise, we're just coming at it from way too many angles. That was really the philosophy that we took.

A lot of it has to do with the board that I have. It's a very strong board. It's a fairly mirrored reflection of our community and a lot of them are actively engaged in our community.

What I think a lot about today is we have a lot of systems that are broken right now in Hawai'i. It's still a beautiful place, but our housing system is broken. We have a lot of work to do in our education system. While the University of Hawai'i leads in many ways there's a lot more that can be done. We should be a globally recognized university. They do a lot. They bring a lot of federal dollars in without a lot of help from many people, including our leaders. So imagine if we could align around the University of Hawai'i, how much it would mean for Hawai'i.

But during a crisis, you have the best opportunity to kind of take off your special interest gloves and dive in for the benefit of the broader good. And I think that's what we saw during the pandemic. A willingness for people to be a lot more vulnerable in their own personal ways and set aside their personal dysfunctions with each other and lay it on the table because it was such a catastrophic hit.

In the past, it was concentrated by geography. You had the Kaua'i floods—that was concentrated on Kaua'i; people in Honolulu and 80 or 90 percent of the elected officials at the state level weren't affected by that. The volcano and the eruptions—again, concentrated within Hawai'i County. This pandemic hit everybody statewide, pretty much equally across the board, because it shut down our biggest industry. And I think that was the fundamental difference. It was as much of an opportunity as it was a challenge.

Kirk Caldwell Chris, you had Peter Ho, Bob Harrison, Paul Yonamine—heads of the largest banks—at the same table sharing their ideas and information even though they are competitors. I've never seen that before.

Chris Benjamin (Alexander & Baldwin) That's one of the great things about Hawai'i. Even in normal times I think we're very collaborative. I sit on the Hawaii Business Roundtable, and Bob Harrison and Peter Ho are right there collaborating even in normal times, and of course in difficult times even more so. The guy that I talked to the most was Peter Ingram because we're friends and I knew that given the nature of his business he was going to be very well versed in these things. I also knew that he was probably more well connected to what was going on than I was. And then the other one was Ray Vara, again for the same reasons. We're friends and with his medical and healthcare perspective he was extremely helpful. So I talked to them a lot, I talked to my internal team of course, and I talked a fair amount to some of the various politicians—you, Derek Kawakami—just to understand the rules as it related to our business operations on the different islands. And then of course, a little bit later, this was probably a few months later, we began to get involved in the tiers.

Bob Harrison, chairman of the board, president, and CEO at First Hawaiian Bank, was about to attend the Hawaii Asia Pacific Association conference in Shanghai when COVID became a concern.

Bob Harrison The first issue at First Hawaiian Bank was our Hawaii Asia Pacific Association trip to Shanghai and inner China in early March. And we're like, *Hey, this doesn't seem like a good idea.* All these business executives, some in their fifties, most in their sixties plus, going to a place of infection, spreading infection, knowing nothing about it and the healthcare system in China. I've never been to mainland China, but the people who have been there said that you don't want to get sick there.

So that was the first discussion. We canceled that trip—I don't even remember when, early on, I think it was still in December or probably early January.

Bob Harrison was also listening to Matt Cox, chairman and CEO of Matson, Inc., whose company runs a thriving shipping service to ports in the People's Republic of China and who was one of the participants that had planned to attend the meeting.

Bob Harrison Well, Matt had people on the ground in Shanghai, which is an important hub for them, and he's been to China dozens of times and just had a feel for it. I don't know if it was a sense—I didn't ask him, but if they're telling you X, it's probably a multiple of X. Maybe that was part of it too, but he was very uncomfortable from the outset and then the rest of us agreed, absolutely. So that was the first thing. Little did we know at the time it was going to grow and turn into a pandemic. Probably by that time, we didn't know it but it had already spread worldwide.

Certainly, in February we were talking about it internally and thinking tourism could clearly be an issue because China was starting to talk very seriously about lockdowns and they had locked down Wuhan and the surrounding area. When you start to see the dominoes starting to teeter, then you know something's up.

In February/early March, when the governor and all the mayors were talking about shutting down, it was clear and the stock market had already gone through a pretty substantial correction and everybody was thinking, *This is a real problem, but no tourism? Nobody going to come? What does that mean for us?*

Iris Ikeda (commissioner of the Hawaii Division of Financial Institutions [DFI]) was doing a good job of getting us together on a regular basis. We were meeting weekly—the CEOs, with her as head of DFI. There was some national communication, not a lot, from the regulators. More state led, at that point, because each state was different so it's not like the federal regulator could come out and say do this for everybody. You really have to respond on a state-by-state basis.

Paul Yonamine, chairman and CEO of Central Pacific Financial Corp., the parent company of Central Pacific Bank, has extensive experience working in Asia. He served as president and country general manager of IBM Japan, Ltd. and is currently board chair of the US-Japan Council.

Paul Yonamine I went through SARS when I was in Japan, when I was with KPMG Consulting, at which point I also oversaw some of our offices in China. That was a scary mini pandemic of sorts, but it was essentially contained within Greater China. Even as recently as February 2020, when I was actually in Japan, I thought that this situation was going to blow over. SARS was really bad but somehow it went away. Or at least it didn't get a lot worse.

I remember being in Tokyo at the time, and then Okinawa, and people were wearing masks, but it was hard to tell if they were wearing masks because of COVID or because of allergies or something else, so I was still under the impression that the outbreak would blow away. But then I came back to Hawai'i in March, and then the governor called the quarantine on March 26, which is when it really hit me. The quarantine meant, besides the health issues, effectively stopping the economy: a seventeen- or eighteen-billion-dollar tourism industry coming to a screeching halt. That economic impact was a big concern for me, for the bank, and for the livelihoods of our employees.

And then on a personal basis, the following day, March 27, my wife's half-brother died. His was the first death from COVID in Oregon. And while I went to his funeral about two months ago, when it was finally possible to have in person, that death made the pandemic very personal at the time even though it was in Oregon. So that's when I think I really realized—March 26 or 27—that this change was very real. And naturally the media was all over the global situation too. Hawai'i was still in a good place then compared to what was happening in Europe, especially Italy, and then in New York, but that's when it really started to set in for me.

Duane Kurisu is the chairman of the board, CEO, and owner of aio, LLC. aio is a holding company for brands in Hawai'i and the Pacific in the areas of media, sports, and food. He also heads the Hawai'i Executive Collaborative, a group of leaders collectively committed to making Hawai'i a better place and to taking responsibility for the future of the Islands. Duane has not only spearheaded this effort, but also organizes the annual Hawai'i Executive Conference.

Duane Kurisu The HEC is a nonprofit organization that works with Hawai'i's leaders in business, government, labor, education, and the community to collaborate in finding solutions and producing tangible results in addressing Hawai'i's most pressing issues. The organization prides itself on being action oriented. It was therefore natural for us to be active in trying to help Hawai'i find its way during the pandemic in 2020. With all of our fears, anxieties, uncertainties, and complexities early on in the pandemic, little could be done without the authority of government, and so we felt that we needed to surround a person with that authority who exhibited leadership and a willingness to try new things. We immediately turned to you, Mayor, and asked if we could surround you and see if you were willing to work together with us to discreetly help Honolulu, and ultimately Hawai'i, have the best chance of seeing its way through COVID-19 and getting on its feet safely and in measured ways.

After working with you, we found that we hadn't been wrong in our judgment about you. Through your leadership, we put together a group of leaders, friends and competitors alike, to talk freely and uninhibitedly about proposing out-of-the-box solutions. We decided to meet weekly to discuss the social and economic climate, what government was doing, how we could provide solutions to help address things and be accountable for what we promised we would do.

Things were constantly changing, and those were scary and stressful times. Thank goodness for Ray Vara of Hawai'i Pacific Health, who provided countless hours of analysis and guidance in helping us understand the COVID environment as best as we could, and for coming up with metrics to help us navigate through uncharted territory. While we weren't always on the same page with you, you had a willingness to try new things, and we almost always, at the end, stood unified on where we stood and where we were going forward.

An example was when you had these federal monies coming, and we talked about where you think the money was going to go and how it was going to be spent. When you presented the idea for a program to give $5,000 to businesses, a bunch of us, myself included, said that amount was not enough. However, after considerable debate, we all agreed it was a good start.

The question then arose, *Who will underwrite the grants and who can quickly and efficiently distribute the money?* Because all the major banks were represented by committee members: Peter Ho, CEO of Bank of Hawai'i; Bob Harrison, CEO of First Hawaiian Bank; Paul Yonamine,

CEO of Central Pacific Bank; and Rich Wacker, CEO of American Savings Bank. And their banks were already involved with the underwriting and distribution of Paycheck Protection Program (PPP) funds. We suggested that it was appropriate that we ask the credit unions. They already represent communities throughout O'ahu and almost all of them weren't previously invited to participate in the PPP programs. I then called on Andy Rosen, president and CEO of Hawaii State Federal Credit Union, who immediately said yes and rounded up the O'ahu credit unions.

In rapid succession, almost all the credit unions committed to be involved. It reminded us of how much Hawai'i is a special place, as the credit union management and staff quickly mobilized to be there for small businesses to apply whether they were credit union customers or not. They rolled up their sleeves to underwrite the huge volume of grants to help the City get the money out. And, Kirk, it's amazing how much money you got out in such a short period of time. In crisis, when people's survival was at stake, it's stunning how things can happen quickly and with such decisiveness when you work within an environment of trust and collaboration. This was truly public-private partnerships working at its best. It's a testament to your leadership. This was just one example of a number of different things that we did together within the committee during the most critical time for Hawai'i.

Other examples where the business community and the Collaborative quietly created important programs with you and the City and County of Honolulu included the inception of:

- The Tier System led by Chris Benjamin, CEO of Alexander & Baldwin; Tina Yamaki, president of the Retail Merchants of Hawaii; Sheryl Matsuoka, executive director of the Hawai'i Restaurant Association; and many industry owners and managers who worked tirelessly to create guidelines to build an environment for the safety of customers and their workers. And in that process, building a tiered system as core to a reopening strategy for Hawai'i.

- The Movers and Shakas program led by Jason Higa, CEO of Zippy's, to attract remote workers and cultivate local style in the way they live, work, and play in Hawai'i.

- The AlohaSafe Alert contact tracing app—an aio Digital-led collaboration with the DOH, which made this Apple and Google platform the most successful digital contact tracing app in the nation.

- The TRUE initiative—brainchild of Paul Yonamine, CEO of Central Pacific Bank, and the Department of Business, Economic Development and Tourism to build awareness and collaboration for companies in Hawai'i to focus on technology as core to their future.

The HEC evolved from its beginning in 1963, when its nonprofit subsidiary, the Hawai'i Executive Conference, was created for networking in business, mostly with executives from the old Big Five companies. When our nonprofit took it over, we saw the need to include leaders in government, labor, education, and the community so that everyone could be in alignment with a collaborative vision and in planning for action and executing on those plans to fulfill that vision.

It was something that kind of evolved quite quickly, especially during the beginning stages of the COVID-19 crisis. We decided along the way that we, as community leaders, should take initiative to be a catalyst for new ideas to solve community issues rather than wait for government to take the lead. While we need government to be a partner, we all felt the need to take responsibility and be accountable for those things that needed innovation and risk-taking and immediate action.

At the same time, local independent schools were also forming their own hui.

Tim Cottrell ('Iolani School) The heads of school—we talked about it. This was back in March 2020 when the impacts of the pandemic were still uncertain. It was starting to brew. The pandemic was starting up with the virus gaining momentum and so we formed a hui with the leaders of the four largest independent schools. The goal was to implement policies and procedures that would have a degree of consistency across schools. The hope was this would make it easier for us to manage what was going on situationally and share information. We were very open source about everything.

As you might expect, everybody came up with their own plan to suit the conditions of their campus. During the summer, we were the first to start talking about coming back. I shared that we were going to return on campus and everyone was going to wear face masks and face shields all the time, and it was greeted with a bit of laughter. I think the general sentiment was that "'Iolani will be out there on this extreme and we will see what happens." But we were very committed to getting our students back on campus as soon as we felt we could do so in a safe way regardless of the practices we needed to mandate. We knew it was vital for the social-emotional health of our students as well as their education.

Dr. David Derauf is not only a medical doctor and public health specialist, but he has also been building a stronger community in Kalihi Valley through improving the health of our most vulnerable populations, such as Pacific Islanders. He has been the executive director of Kōkua Kalihi Valley since 1989. During the onset of COVID, the Pacific Islander community was the hardest hit of all ethnic groups. He served on the mayor's advisory panel for COVID, and his candid assessment on policy and operations, how we were doing, and what we should be doing was invaluable.

David Derauf I was on my last vacation, the very last vacation I took before the pandemic hit Hawai'i. I was up in northern Wisconsin in a cabin in the woods and checking my email. This would have been the end of December. In this cabin with a roaring fire, a long way away, it seemed hard to imagine that this was coming our way. But I really did have a gut feeling that something wasn't right. Unlike prior times when we had had some warning signs that such and such virus was spreading a bit, I never really got nervous, but something hit me in my gut with this one.

January 3, I sent off an email to the DOH epidemiologist, saying I'm increasingly worried about what we're seeing here. What assessment had been made of the risk to Hawai'i? What preparations were being made? The answer I received back concerned me: *We don't have anything to worry about. We don't have direct flights from China*. And that's when I first got really worried. Events continued to unfold as we know them now.

The other part of it was the CDC. People didn't really realize that the sort of international playbook for epidemic management that the CDC had subscribed to really didn't believe in cutting off transportation to China or any other place as part of pandemic management, nor really in quarantine and isolation. They didn't initially believe, as we know, in masks. So, the response of DOH in that sense really was following the playbook that was standard to CDC. Maybe that wasn't such a good idea, but at the time they thought that was the established dogma. I think a lot of that will be challenged going forward and we'll be fighting over these decisions for years to come.

It's really one of the sadder things for all of us who have had careers in public health that this once world-renowned institution, the CDC, literally was where all the best people in the world had gone to get trained. The best people from China, Thailand, Vietnam—they were all trained there, and yet they've let everyone down time and time again during this pandemic by frequent dramatic shifts in messaging and guidance. Don't mask, do mask, etc. The institution itself feels broken and that is a sad thing to say. Many, many good people have left. However, that happened. The institution is not a strong institution and we badly needed a strong institution.

For my part, Jon Dworkin and I ended up at one of the first statewide COVID response meetings. A large group of people were there representing the hospitals, public health institutions. I was there representing community health centers.

I guess I had hoped that out of that meeting there would be a real division of labor. We could say, "Who's interested in isolation and quarantine? Who's interested in public health messaging? Who's interested in vaccine deployment? Who on testing protocols?" And all that. I thought we could organize, we could break it up. There's tons of smart people;

there's no shortage of smarts. I'm looking around the room, we've got so much intelligence there, it seems we could solve any problem.

But it seemed to me that our emergency preparations had not ever focused on how we cooperate. How do we self-organize quickly? How do we break this down into bite-sized pieces? And how do we protect our most vulnerable communities like Kalihi? So, what ended up happening was every institution was pretty much left to their own. *You figure out what you're going to do for testing. You figure out what you're going to do for masking.* It wasn't formally said, but Jon and I looked at each other. I knew him a little bit already, and we looked at each other alarmed.

This was like in March. We knew it was coming at this point and as an organization we were starting to prepare. And I think we knew enough about DOH and their capacity to know that they were going to need help. ✻

CHAPTER 2

Lockdown

Nine days after the first COVID case in Hawai'i, Ray Vara, Peter Ho, and Micah Kane talked early in the morning and decided they had to go see the governor as soon as possible. Their data showed that unless action was taken soon, the exponential growth of the virus would devastate the state. It was March 15, a Sunday morning, but the matter was urgent.

Ray Vara (Hawai'i Pacific Health) Peter Ho and I were talking early in the morning and decided that we should go visit the governor. So we reached out to the governor's office that morning, March 15, and asked if we could come see him. They said yes, if we could be there by 11 a.m. We also reached out to Micah Kane to join us. We were in shorts and T-shirts as we went into the governor's conference room.

Governor Ige, Maj. Gen. Ken Hara, Linda Chu Takayama, Bruce Anderson, and others from his staff were all there. They were working to figure out the appropriate next steps. We expressed that we believed it was time to start shutting things down. Close the schools, limit gatherings, close restaurants, close bars... It's just time to start winding things down. The quicker we act, the better this will be. The governor was on the phone with the DOE leadership at the time. That's when they decided they were going to extend spring break by four days.

We had hoped for a more aggressive response.

Peter Ho (Bank of Hawai'i) I remember saying to the governor, "You know, we're here to support you, but we think you need to do something. Wouldn't you agree?" And it was like, "Yeah, we know we need to do something, but we don't know what to do." And we started laying out what we would do if asked. An early thought was that we really need to stand up our public health capability. We started talking about the concept of contact tracing. Testing—although come to find out later that that just didn't exist, right? Even if we wanted to, it didn't exist. But contact tracing, which interestingly became an early political ping-pong ball, it just kind of fell on deaf ears.

That was Sunday. We were very direct with him. *Look, you gotta do this, this, this, and this. The quicker we act, the quicker we shut this thing down.* We felt we didn't get as much coming out of that as we would have liked because he was only talking about deciding whether he was going to extend spring break. That was it.

We asked Governor David Ige if he remembered the meeting on March 15 and what he was thinking at the time about a possible shutdown.

David Ige It was a couple of different things. I was aware that they really felt that more direct action had to be taken. But I also believe that it had to be something that we coordinated with the counties. There's a couple of things—and it goes back to even the quarantine issue. It's easy to order something; it's hard to implement in a way that is workable. And so certainly I did understand what the impact of stay-at-home orders or quarantine orders would be on our economy. And I did want to make sure that it was the right decision to make. It is one of those things that I've been criticized for, not responding quick enough, but I do think in hindsight that it was the right decision to be made in a lot of different ways.

I grew up on the notion that if you don't have something good to say about someone, you shouldn't comment. I still have a hard time criticizing people publicly. I think part of the issue, when I had talked with other mayors, they weren't at the point that they wanted to shut down. I think we all understood what would happen and the statewide stay-at-home order for all of the counties, they were not at the same place that you, Mayor, were. And the question was whether it would be ordered on like Kaua'i, very rural—it's not the same kind of place as Honolulu. That's the challenge: Do you impose it on everybody regardless of what they think or do you allow some flexibility?

Ray Vara sent a graph depicting the projected spread of the virus to Mayor Caldwell in the following days.

Ray Vara (Hawai'i Pacific Health) I think it was the following Saturday and we were continuing to get more concerned at the pace in which things were moving. That is when we reached out to you, Mayor. You were obviously trying to get out in front of this, and I believe had you not jumped into action the situation could have gotten much worse very quickly.

Micah Kane (Hawai'i Community Foundation) The governor gave us an audience, which was important. When we realized that we weren't going to get traction there, we tactically decided that we were going to take it down to the next highest level of government. That's when we ended up with Kirk Caldwell. And the fact that he opened his door to us and was willing to stay engaged and to get more data, more information, willing to try to understand what the lay of the land was—that was a big difference. Having the 800-pound gorilla of our state, the largest of the four counties, realize that that leadership was going to have to come at that level—that was important.

Like Alexander & Baldwin, Peter Ho could not and did not wait for a government order to take action at the Bank of Hawai'i.

Peter Ho The health and safety of our employees and our customers were paramount. But the practical reality is that the fastest way to get the economy back on trajectory is to get the health situation taken care of, and until you do it doesn't matter what you do because people are pretty smart and they are going to be looking out for the most fundamental need, which is safety and shelter, before they go out and spend money. I mean, maybe bars will be the exception because they'd all be commiserating in the bar, but they won't be at Ala Moana Center shopping, right?

Kirk Caldwell Not all businesses took a strong, lean forward, public position like you did. Under your leadership, Bank of Hawai'i very early on took strong measures to protect your employees and your customers before a lot of other institutions. You were careful. You wanted to make sure that everyone was safe. And you implemented all kinds of initiatives from working from home to handing out meals to your employees—those types of things. You had the macro vision and then you had a very specific micro vision for your institution.

Peter Ho As a public corporation, we have all these different stakeholders. We have customers, employees, shareholders, regulators, and the art of managing is understanding that sometimes certain stakeholders have to come ahead of others. And if you get that sequencing right, more times than not, ultimately you've got a chance to be successful.

I think it might have been a day or so after you and I were chatting, I spoke to Mike O'Neill (former president and CEO of Bank of Hawai'i) and he said, "Yeah this is not good. This is a situation where the shareholders are going to take a second seat to the interests of other stakeholders because it's just going to be one of these things." And that in part helped shape my thinking, which was that the bank's got plenty of capital and the best way to protect our shareholders is to make sure that we're protecting the assets that are most important to our shareholders long term, which are our customers and employees. The human capital.

And it just was kind of obvious, so we sent people home a week before the state mandate.

Around the same time, March 15, Peter Ingram at Hawaiian Airlines had started planning for a possible travel shutdown.

Peter Ingram We had started planning for how we would spool down the flying of the airline because at the time there was talk of the coming pandemic having a major impact on the airline industry. I got back from Washington, DC, that weekend of the 9th. The next week, the NCAA tournament got canceled. It was in the middle of the afternoon. I was in a meeting with my officer team and before the meeting ended the NBA suspended their season. In addition, it was announced that Tom Hanks had COVID in Australia. It was all in one meeting. We were sitting upstairs and it was like this stuff was just coming rapid fire now. These events are sort of pop culture important, but it was just showing how pervasive this was getting.

We started hearing rumors for the airline industry that there may be a call to ground flying for a couple of weeks nationwide to stop the spread, and it turns out that that was never seriously on the table. But we didn't know if those rumors were rooted in some reality, so we spent a weekend with a small group secretly building a plan for what we would do if we had to ground the airline. Where do we put the airplanes? How do we get crews back?

I was working in the airline industry at American Airlines during 9/11. It was a different sort of shutdown in that there was no notice. No planes could enter the country and anything in the air was ordered to land ASAP, so you ended up with planes and crews all in wrong places. We assumed with something like this (COVID), because we were flying safely at that point, that there would be at least forty-eight-hours' notice. So, we started building a plan that laid out what we would do if we had forty-eight hours to grind everything to a halt. How do we get all of the crews back to where they need to be? How do we get any crew members who live in Hawai'i back to Hawai'i, and crew members who live on the Mainland back to the Mainland? How do we take our guests home from their trips? And that plan ended up, ten days later, to be the bones of what we implemented when the quarantine went into effect.

So we had a plan of winding it down, trying to make sure there were enough flights back to the Mainland even if they were going to be empty coming back over here, so if people were on vacation over here they had a chance to get out before we started canceling everything. We pretty quickly implemented it over about a five-day period. We ended up stretching it out because we didn't have the two-day constraint, but we wound our schedule down.

The Honolulu mayor held a press conference on Thursday, March 19,

2020, to announce the restaurant shutdown—takeout only, effective Friday, March 20, 2020, at 8:30 a.m.

Kirk Caldwell By the second week in March, we shut down all restaurants on O'ahu except for takeout. We were the first government entity in the state of Hawai'i to do that, and we did that because we were reading that restaurants were a source of spreading the virus.

It's no secret that one of Kirk's favorite places to eat is Zippy's. We interviewed Jason Higa (CEO) and Paul Yokota (president) of FCH Enterprises, the parent company of Zippy's, named after Francis and Charlie Higa, brothers and co-founders. We asked about the origin of the name Zippy's. Jason explained that the business was formed in 1966, a few years after the zip code was created and highly promoted in 1963 by the US Postal Service. Francis and Charlie thought of the name Zippy's after the name Zip's could not be registered.

Paul Yokota As a company, we were fortunate because we have multiple concepts. We have our fast-food concept as well as our dine-in concept. So when dine-in had to shut down in March 2020, we still had our fast-food operation. Our dine-in food inventories were shifted to our fast-food operation and many staff shifted as well.

Due to the closure of our dine-in operations and reduction in operating hours, our human resources department fielded many calls regarding concerns from our employees. We did our best to address as many issues as possible immediately. We had fortunately developed a paid time off program prior to the pandemic, allowing employees, who were subject to reduced schedules, to take the paid time off to subsidize their income. There were calls on benefits, unemployment insurance, and schedules. Unfortunately, certain operations had to be shuttered. As our dine-in operations were closed, many of our dine-in employees were offered positions in our fast-food operations.

In the early months of the pandemic, many employees chose not to work because of the concerns with contracting COVID. Therefore, we had to determine how to operate with limited staffing. Certain locations were closed, others reduced operating hours, and new services like curbside pickup were created. Many of our wait help staff, for example, helped with our fast-food curbside service.

For our catering operation, A Catered Experience, we could no longer operate at the Hawaii Okinawa Center and our Pomaika'i Ballrooms and, unfortunately, were forced to shut down permanently.

We adjusted our administrative offices to allow for working from home. We determined who could work remotely and who needed to come to the office.

Kirk Caldwell I remember when restaurants were shut, I would come to Zippy's Makiki a lot because it's halfway between our home and work, and it felt safe getting takeout from you guys. When this happened, did you think this was going to last for a while or did you think you would be back to dine-in in a couple of weeks?

Paul Yokota We had been through other crises. We survived the 2008 Great Recession. We have also been through earthquakes, tsunami warnings, and hurricanes. So we initially applied our existing emergency protocols for temporarily reducing operations. However, the pandemic was far different and required us to adapt quite a bit.

Jason Higa We were just doing things, I hate to say it, day-to-day. Things were changing so quickly, and Paul, along with our operations team, did a great job making the appropriate adjustments along the way.

Kirk Caldwell To me, you got organized quickly. The use of plexiglass between tables, the placing of the footprints on the floor for physical distancing, the placing of a table in front of the counter to create more space between the customer and the cashier. Later, the temperature taking, the emailing of your customers in their cars to let them know when their orders were ready, and the delivering of food to your customers' cars. You tapped into some strong and unique COVID protocols.

Georgette Deemer (author) The thing that I thought was genius was that you also were selling toilet paper. And I thought, *OMG, okay, maybe I don't need Zippy's chili, but I really need that toilet paper, so I'm going to go to Zippy's!*

Paul Yokota As you may recall, people were concerned about going out, period, especially to crowded places like supermarkets. We thought if they're coming to Zippy's let's have necessities available to them so they don't have to make a second trip elsewhere. That is where toilet paper and other items like yeast were offered for sale.

Georgette Deemer Yes, the yeast! Because there was this baking run on flour and yeast. Everyone was home making banana bread and sourdough. The shelves were empty at the store.

Paul Yokota Our marketing team monitored social media platforms to determine which items were in short supply, our operations team monitored what COVID protocols were being adopted by the restaurant industry, and our human resources team worked closely with the DOH on close contact reporting and other mandated protocols. We formed the Zip Team—forgive the name—to develop and implement new concepts quickly. Our mantra became "survive to thrive" (i.e., survive today so we can thrive tomorrow). Move quickly on what we need to do, what we have to change, to be ahead of the curve. No idea was a bad idea. We put everything on the table.

Jason Higa Early on, we decided that we were going to make fast decisions at the expense of making thoughtful decisions, which would take longer. Things were just moving so quickly. If a decision had merit, we did it and awaited the results. If it worked out, great, and if it didn't work, we could just change.

Kirk Caldwell Initially, we closed restaurants except for takeout. We followed San Francisco's order. About a week later we announced the full O'ahu lockdown. How did this impact your takeout business?

Paul Yokota Our fast-food operations were steady. Sales were far below what we normally did, but it was steady because customers were still craving our menu items as comfort food. The drop in sales was also location dependent. For example, our downtown locations had a significant drop in sales as most downtown offices closed. However, locations outside of the city saw smaller reductions.

In the days following the restaurant shutdown, the City heard from the community on some critical impacts, such as the need for hospital food services to remain open, and modifications were immediately made. But the most serious lockdown was soon to come. On Saturday, March 21, 2020, Mayor Caldwell met with Governor Ige to inform him that the City had prepared a lockdown order based on a model recently implemented by the city of San Francisco. He wanted the governor to consider a statewide lockdown and to join with him on the announcement.

Kirk Caldwell We went over and Bruce Anderson—the director of health—was there. The governor's chief of staff was there. A couple other people too. And we told him that we want to issue a work-from-home, stay-at-home order modeled after San Francisco—we think it's the right thing to do.

Bruce Anderson dominated the conversation. The governor listens a lot; he doesn't talk so much. Anderson said, "There's pukas here that you could drive a Mack truck through. Look, you made construction workers essential workers. You made grocery stores essential." That was because people need to eat and construction is the third largest industry in the state of Hawai'i, and without tourism it would become the second largest industry after the military. In addition, construction work was mostly done in open spaces where masks are required. We didn't come up with this without a lot of thought and it was based on the San Francisco stay-at-home, work-from-home order, which was considered a very strong model for combating the virus. But Bruce was against it. We spent maybe two hours, from about 3 to 5 p.m., talking about it. And then at 5:00, because I knew we had a lot of remaining work to do, I told the governor, "You know we came over here not to ask for your permission, because we don't have to. But I was hoping that you would join us and make this a statewide order, an order for everyone, and that we would go together."

He didn't say yes or no, but I said, "We're going to do it." So we went back to Honolulu Hale and began finalizing all the necessary steps to implement the order.

I thought it was the right thing. I still think it was the correct action to take at the time. I just wish we could have done it together.

Leading up to the meeting with the governor, I had the growing feeling that we needed to do more. There was a small but increasing number of cases on O'ahu. But what really tipped it for me was earlier that same day Peter Ho and Ray Vara called me up and said, "We have some information that you'll find very interesting and very disturbing. Can we send it to you?" I said, "Yes, send it now." What was sent to me was data from Pierre Omidyar's Hawaii Data Collaborative. The Hawaii Data Collaborative analyzed data on COVID cases on O'ahu and in the state of Hawai'i and made some projections on the future growth of cases if no action was taken. It showed that from March to May our hospitals would be overwhelmed with patients and people could be dying in the corridors of hospitals if we didn't act. We figured Omidyar is a smart guy. He has smart guys working for him. His information was verified and supported by Ray Vara's HPH data people. There were graphs and numbers, just three or four pages, nicely laid out, and it screamed out for action.

The next day, which was Sunday, we held a press conference in the atrium of the Hale to ensure better social distancing. We announced we're going to be locking down the island of O'ahu starting at 4:30 p.m. on Monday. We selected 4:30 based on Peter Ho's advice that it would give businesses at least twenty-four hours advance notice to prepare for the lockdown. This would give them time to notify their employees and to deal with products with limited shelf life.

On that Tuesday morning around 3 a.m., after the lockdown went into effect, I got up and looked across Mānoa Valley where I live and there was just silence. Not a car was on the road. I thought about the impact this was going to have for everyone on O'ahu. People weren't going to go to work tomorrow, people were scared, and no one knew if this lockdown was going to last two weeks, one month, or longer but I just knew it was going to have major impact.

As the mayor, as the person at the top of the pyramid, you make the decision and you live with the decision. It can be very lonely, but it comes with the job.

Dennis Francis (Oahu Publications) I had just seen the report from San Francisco where the mayor was shutting down the city, sending everybody but essential workers home—like a major storm was coming. And I have lived in Hawai'i long enough to know that when anything major like this impacts the Mainland, it eventually hits us here in Hawai'i. So when the lockdown was given for San Francisco, I knew this was coming our way too.

Kirk Caldwell Dennis, you suggested that we should consider a lockdown order like San Francisco. This would have a direct negative impact on your paper from a revenue perspective, and yet you suggested it. I call that leadership. Did you think about the consequences at the time you were suggesting that we take such action?

Dennis Francis Yes and no. The first reaction is about safety. You want to make sure your people are safe. So I really wasn't thinking about the impact to our business. And it soon became clear that a lockdown eventually was going to happen. I thought we might as well get ahead of the curve and be safe. It's inevitable, so better early than later.

Kirk Caldwell So you put your readers' health ahead of business.

Dennis Francis Yeah, basically our employees, our readers, and the entire community. I thought that the lockdown was critical, and in retrospect it was clearly the right call. The lockdowns weren't an answer to everything, but they did help lessen the damage.

Kirk Caldwell I remember on the day of the lockdown your headline read LOCKDOWN in four-inch high letters. Everyone's lives on O'ahu were affected, including your workforce.

Dennis Francis Before the pandemic we had about 425 employees, and today we have about 325. So we lost about a hundred people.

Kirk Caldwell Pre-pandemic, journalists and others would go into your newsroom, close together, and now you're trying to manage a paper and a workforce that is no longer coming to work.

Dennis Francis That was one of the first things we did. We qualified as essential workers and we still had to publish. We obviously didn't want people to come to work sick, so we immediately had almost everyone work from home, with a skeleton crew in the newsroom, mainly some editors. I came in every single day from day one of the pandemic. I was in the office every day. And we published every day. To this day, most of those employees who were assigned to work from home at the start of the pandemic are still doing so.

It's one of those interesting things in a union environment. Before the pandemic, the union would occasionally request the ability to work from home and I was adamant about not allowing this—we can't control that, we don't know what they're doing, and so forth. But what the pandemic showed me was that this was wrong. People can be productive and do a lot of the work that they need to do from home. In some cases, they are even more productive because they have more flexibility to take care of personal issues, such as child care.

EDUCATION LOCKDOWN

David Ige (Governor of Hawai'i) We were all struggling. I think we all naively thought that if we shut down that things would be resolved relatively quickly. They're on spring break, maybe we can extend the break, for a week, maybe a couple weeks. But you know, my expectation was that we would reopen, that we would be able to contain the virus, that we would reopen clearly before the end of the school year and get caught up.

We did think about what that would mean from a contract perspective. Obviously, we knew that we would incur costs, but what can we do if we did take a break to make sure the kids could catch up? I certainly didn't think that at that point in time it would be a shutdown for the rest of the year. I thought we would get the virus under control and that we would reopen the schools.

Christina Kishimoto, superintendent of the DOE, provided the following statistics: A shutdown of the public schools would impact 180,000 children, including charter school kids; 13,000 teachers; 40,000 employees.

Christina Kishimoto By the end of March, first week of April, we decided to shut down for the rest of the school year.

Kirk Caldwell You're announcing this, and parents and students are wondering what's going to happen. How are kids going to learn? And you've got teachers and employees, everyone: *Do I come to work? What do I do?* How did you manage all of this?

Christina Kishimoto Everyone wanted a clear playbook, instantly, and that wasn't possible. We needed to design this as we went and figure out exactly what we needed to make decisions on. And so I set up an emergency response team immediately and we set up a daily meeting, and then with my complex area superintendents, meetings twice a week, and we called more meetings as necessary. And we did that for almost an entire year.

Kirk Caldwell Complex area superintendents from the Neighbor Islands were on this call too?

Christina Kishimoto Yes, talking together, saying, "When the superintendent is sending a message out, what is that going to mean?" We gave it to them first so that when the message went out there was a whole team ready to answer questions. Otherwise everything was going to come to my office and there's no way I could manage that. So we ended up with fifteen complex area superintendents and seven assistant superintendents all standing by to handle different components of the employee groups and parents to answer questions.

Kirk Caldwell You also implemented a robust food distribution program for children who were no longer coming to school but prior to that were depending on the public school system for at least one decent meal a day. How did you implement this program?

Christina Kishimoto We stood up meal service almost immediately in April. We don't usually distribute food during spring break. In April, we had to prepare our staff to get all the PPE to be able to hand out meals, and I give them a lot of credit. I didn't have any food service team members or volunteers tell me, "No, I'm not going to feed." We got permission from the USDA right away to feed anyone under the age of eighteen, which meant that we got into our summer feeding allotment. They needed to work quickly and I didn't have funds for this either so by midyear I'm $24 million in the hole doing a feeding program for kids across the entire state.

We ran into challenges that needed to be solved, such as, *Well, if I'm not going to school why would I go there to pick up a meal?* Okay, so what do we do? We know who our kids in crisis are, so we literally were loading up vans and dropping off food to our kids in crisis.

Kirk Caldwell You would go to their homes?

Christina Kishimoto We did this very quietly and we got USDA permission for it, but I wasn't going to seek a bunch of permission here to try to feed kids. In addition to school sites, we pushed this out through vans. For our homeless students, we loaded up vans with a Yes bus, so they could visibly see us coming. We put new decals on buses, drove them to different locations to drop off to our homeless students that we knew where they were, and that went really well. Once people started feeling comfortable coming out, then the issue became *I don't want to* *come out twice, once for breakfast once for lunch.* So we got permission again from USDA to package breakfast and lunch together for one pickup. And we also got permission to be able to have a family come through, show us the IDs of their children and be able to pick up the meals for their children. We fed both public and private school children.

The complexity is not just the logistics, the operational logistics, but we're running under state and federal laws, and when you're handling food, just that alone is complex. And we were out of money. Basically, what I said was I'm not going to stop feeding kids. I didn't have money and I didn't have answers from anyone, despite repeatedly asking whether I should be overspending in this area, but I thought if anything we're going to figure out internally how to pay this off. For this, I'm going to figure it out.

Kirk Caldwell The food distribution program that you implemented is so heartrending. I remember watching the news stories and seeing these families driving up, getting meals for their kids. Their parents had lost their jobs, they had no income. So now at least their kids are getting meals. As a parent, you're worried about being able to feed your family, but at least the school system is helping you do that. This is a very powerful story.

Christina Kishimoto We did things in real time everywhere we could to address the needs of our schools. We worked with the Hawai'i Emergency Management Agency (HI-EMA), but they would only drop off pallets of PPE, and now I'm in one room, one gymnasium of a high school, filled floor to ceiling with PPE for the entire state, nearly three hundred schools, and I've got to break down pallets. None of us do this for a living. We got together with a team. HI-EMA stepped in at one point, helped us out. We had banks of volunteers. And when I say volunteers I'm talking about my team, my employees—they're just coming out. We outfitted them with PPE, they're breaking down pallets, and packaging per school, per island, per complex, and then figuring out who's going to ship this. It was an unbelievable operational nightmare. And thankfully HI-EMA stepped in after seeing the nightmare we were trying to handle and took over getting everything to the other islands. That was a huge help for us.

Logistically, we're calling our partners, asking them, "Hey, you got a truck going over there? You got a boat going over there? You got a barge? You got a plane going over there?" You know, again, we're not one landmass and just the logistics of this was really hard.

A whole bunch of issues just piled up. We're trying to answer things around *How are you instructing? and Are teachers getting paid for this time? What happens to the custodian who can't come in to clean because the building's shut down? Does that mean he or she's going on some kind of furlough?*

The mayors were great. The governor was great. It didn't mean we were all in agreement in knowing what to do, especially early on, but what was great was being able to say, "Look, the list of things that the superintendent has to make a decision on is just growing exponentially and she can't be everywhere and her team can't be everywhere." We were doing crisis support for families, literally knocking on doors, checking on kids. We have kids who have safety issues and we have to notify people of those issues so we know who they are. We're checking in on children, and we're doing all these things, and you've got to do that confidentially. It's not like you can tell the media I couldn't be there because I'm checking on my list of a couple hundred kids that are on suicide watch, who are in a family in crisis, there's abuse in that family. You just can't talk about those things—and you shouldn't, publicly. So, we're trying to manage that so that we don't have a child that's unsafe.

Kirk Caldwell Are you doing all of this from your office?

Christina Kishimoto I told everyone "jeans and sneakers"—get comfortable because we're going to be running wherever, and it was seven days a week. And it was nonstop for months and months and months. It started in March 2020, and it's insane—it was not till maybe November that any of us are looking up. And at that point I'm concerned about the mental health of my own staff and burnout. I have staff who now have lost a family member from COVID. I have staff who have lost a parent to old age. And they're grieving and they're trying to do this and they can't get on a plane and get back home. We have staff who live in Maui who are trying to work from my office here in Honolulu.

I think the hardest part of the whole pandemic was what it felt like, after a while, a lack of recognition of the complexity of what we were managing. And what I think, at this point in time, this late in the year, what my staff feels is a lack of gratitude for what they did. As a leader, that was really hard—to start noticing that they felt the lack of gratitude.

This staff got together and has become really close. We just had a retirement of someone who has served for over thirty years here in the DOE. He was ready to retire and it's great, but there were tears all around. I mean everyone has just become this close-knit family and they were already close. That's the beautiful part of what comes out of all of our effort, but you also don't want people feeling hurt at the end of this.

Tim Cottrell ('Iolani School) We started planning weeks in advance for a potential shutdown in 2020. We set up the technology, Zoom linked to each student's schedule, and asked our faculty to practice teaching online while still on campus. So our students would sit throughout campus and use their iPads to Zoom into class just like they would if we had to transition online with them at home. We also tested the home Wi-Fi connection of all our families to ensure connectivity would not be a problem. So when we decided to go online it was pretty easy and seamless for us. We had everything in place. We had the technology in place, we had teacher training, and we had student training. As a result, we were ready, and I think we were quite a bit ahead of the curve at this time.

Kirk Caldwell That's impressive.

Tim Cottrell Realistically, this was a little easier for us than most other schools. Both because of our iPad program and timing. I don't really know what happened with the DOE, but with our peer schools, they were on break. So the decision to close on-campus operations happened when they were on break. Schools then needed to bring people back from break, train them, train their students, set up the technology, and do this in real time when they were transitioning to an online program—when students and faculty were no longer on campus. We benefited from doing this work well in advance when people could learn the tools with in-person support and training.

Kirk Caldwell When we announced the stay-at-home, work-from-home order, we did not consult you or others in the education field. Did this make it more difficult for you?

Tim Cottrell I feel that in general there wasn't a lot of cohesive communication going on anywhere, right? It wasn't just the city government or county. There wasn't a lot of direction on the state level, from the DOH, the DOE, and there was misinformation on the federal level, so it was just a big mess and, institutionally, each school was kind of on their own to plan and implement. So we just took it upon ourselves with the understanding that everybody's going to be responsible to make this work for their situation and constituency. That was the main lens for us. We wanted to do our best and as good a job as possible, given the conditions and available information. We made all of our decisions grounded in science, with the needs of our students, faculty, and staff at the forefront, and when we did receive the stay-at-home mandate we were ready.

We also immediately started thinking about how we could use our resources to help the community. We transformed our iLab in the Sullivan Center for Innovation and Leadership into a face shield factory. We had over twenty 3D printers and two laser cutters working around the clock to fabricate over 17,000 face shields. The demand was huge at the time because there was a supply shortage. We gave the shields for free to Hawaiʻi's frontline workers and emergency responders. We also provided face shields to nursing homes, physician offices, teachers—really anyone who emailed us to receive one. We also helped with creating intubation boxes for Hawaiʻi's hospitals and the team in our Sullivan Center wet lab worked in partnership with Dr. Marguerite Butler at the University of Hawaiʻi, and Pamela O'Brien and Edward Desmond from the DOH to find ways we could assist with COVID tracking. To date, using our ʻĀina-Informatics Network curriculum, students across eight schools have safely sequenced 246 deactivated SARS-CoV-2 genomes from real Hawai'i patients, empowering the next generation of epidemiologists, virologists, and crisis managers.

Kirk Caldwell When you did close, the parents were prepared for this because you already were talking to their children about learning online.

Tim Cottrell Yeah, they were already doing it. We had a whole conversation about the dynamic, about how online learning places parents in the role of being quasi-educators. We wanted to be sure they had computers and the necessary bandwidth. We did bandwidth checks in all our families' homes and we provided connections to homes that didn't have good internet bandwidth. Soup to nuts.

I'd say a general theme that worked well for us throughout the whole process was to constantly overcommunicate. We have probably said that word a million times in the last sixteen months. Overcommunicate. Nobody wants surprises. Nobody wants to feel like they don't know what's going on. Everyone might not like the decisions you make, but we needed to create a context for everything that's going on and the decisions being made. We were good that way. Our one-team culture really united us in all we did. It's a culture that our community truly believes in and it allowed us to be united in our efforts to keep everyone safe and provide consistent communication and messaging in the midst of all the noise and disinformation that was going on in the world.

Kirk Caldwell When you made the announcement that 'Iolani was going to online learning from home, what was the reaction among parents and students?

Tim Cottrell We have people in our community who were pretty connected to what was happening in the world. Dr. Mark Mugiishi, CEO of HMSA, is our board chair. Dr. Mugiishi, along with other experts in the medical field, were instrumental in advising us. There wasn't a credibility gap in what we were saying to our families.

We knew this was not going to go away. We had a plan, provided regular updates to our parents, and this ultimately enabled us to gain their trust and community alignment. They were very supportive. We accepted that we were most likely going to be online for the remaining months of the 2020 school year, prepared with this in mind, and I think, ultimately, this helped us a lot over the entire span of the pandemic—establishing trust and alignment right from the start.

David Lassner (University of Hawai'i) As the situation evolved and the numbers increased, we of course got nervous but, more importantly, also got serious. We first decided that we would have to go fully online after spring break. We made that announcement, I believe, as the first major enterprise in Hawai'i to make it clear that our world was about to change. At first we thought we would only have to be online for a couple of weeks after spring break. But the week before spring break started, we realized that the situation was increasingly serious and we publicly announced we would be online for the rest of the semester.

Governor Ige is a strong supporter of UH autonomy and never micromanaged or second-guessed our internal decision-making. Our authority and decision-making regarding our educational and research mission and employment practices were never questioned. Issues around public gatherings like fans at sporting events were broader public health issues over which we followed State and City and County guidance. But we had full authority over how we managed instruction. The executive proclamations generally exempted education, but we kept in touch. Governor Ige includes me in his cabinet, so I was in many of the key conversations about pandemic conditions, state of our healthcare systems, mitigation measures, and the like.

Within UH, we are blessed with significant medical and public health expertise and experience. So we were able to convene our own internal Health and Wellbeing Working Group to give us advice on our guidelines and practices on matters relating to distancing, testing, vaccinations, and all things COVID. Over time, different people have really stepped up in different roles. The associate dean, Lee Buenconsejo-Lum, of the medical school has been awesome. The dean of nursing, Mary Boland, actually delayed her retirement so she could help us through the pandemic. The dean of our medical school, Jerris Hedges, regularly reminded us that we needed to mitigate COVID-19 risks but could not eliminate them entirely without compromising other aspects of public health and well-being. For example, the best way to stop the spread of COVID would have been to keep everybody home. But that would have had consequences around matters such as economic well-being and food security of families not working, mental health under total isolation, and loss of opportunity for students unable to complete their higher education to create better futures for themselves. It was not about one hundred percent guarantees against COVID, but balancing risks.

Kirk Caldwell Did the regents weigh in?

David Lassner I briefed the regents regularly at their monthly meetings and consulted on major decisions in advance. They've been really good about recognizing their role as a governing board and leaving the administration to manage the crisis day-to-day and month-to-month.

Kirk Caldwell Our first stay-at-home, work-from-home order, which went into effect the third week of March, didn't have much impact on you because you had already made a decision not to return to in-school classroom learning, correct?

David Lassner That's right. And education was exempt in the executive proclamations, in part because the governor saw that we were already proactive and managing ourselves. Our principle in those early days was to draw a bright line that said if something can only be done in person you can do it and these are the protocols. Lab and studio courses would be a good example of this, along with shop classes in career and technical education, and of course clinical experiences in the health sciences. We wanted to ensure our students could stay on track toward graduation in whatever they studied. And we went remote for what we could—lecture and discussion sections of courses.

One key decision we made was to allow students living in our residence halls to stay on campus. It would have been "safer" for us to close our residences, but many of those students would have nowhere to go and campus was the safest place for them.

We spent that whole spring break helping our faculty prepare to teach online, upgrading our IT systems to scale up to support every class across our campuses, physically distancing our classrooms, developing cleaning procedures, preparing quarantine and isolation protocols including contracting with a hotel, which was easy then since hotels were largely vacant.

Our faculty were amazing at pulling off the immediate and unexpected shift online and our students adapted incredibly well. Most students here, even if they're living on campus, take an online class or two anyway. We have many online classes and some students just enjoy that mode of instruction. So we had the tools in place already so that every UH course on every campus had an online presence even if the only content might be the syllabus and grades. The shell was all there, the software was all there, and most faculty knew how to use our system and they were fantastic in helping each other. Our chief information officer, who has my former job, and our IT team were remarkable in scaling everything up by a factor of ten or more, but the pieces were all there.

Kirk Caldwell You run a statewide system. Did your response or actions differ by county?

David Lassner We made all major decisions as a system, but they were implemented locally. So we didn't decide as a system which classes were absolutely required to be in person. But we said that if the class has to be in person, then you've got to do physical distancing. But we are pretty system-oriented in our thinking and planning, so our policies, guidelines, software, and tools were all systemwide.

Kirk Caldwell Did the student body, depending on what island you were on, have challenges regarding connectivity?

David Lassner I don't think it was so much by island, but we definitely had students throughout the state with connectivity challenges.

We used some of our federal relief funds to set up pools of loaner equipment. Students could check out laptops and Wi-Fi hot spots from our libraries. And some students drove to campus to use Wi-Fi from their cars in parking lots.

TRAVEL AND THE FOURTEEN-DAY QUARANTINE

Kirk Caldwell The decision on the fourteen-day quarantine for everyone coming into Hawai'i was historic. Never done by any other state. Is that correct?

David Ige (Governor of Hawai'i) Other states did order a quarantine, but nobody did anything to implement it. In all the other states, I know in that March and April time frame when I looked on the states, I think about twenty to twenty-three states had ordered quarantine for incoming travelers but nobody actually enforced their quarantines.

Kirk Caldwell It can be difficult to enforce a quarantine on the New Jersey Turnpike.

David Ige Right, and you knew and I knew that if we ordered the quarantine and we talked about it, it had to mean something. I wasn't just going to order a quarantine like the other states and do nothing about it. And if we did order the quarantine, we knew that we would effectively shut down travel. I didn't think that it would be 99.9 percent effective. If I sat and thought about it, I would come to that conclusion. We thought that we would definitely have an impact on travel, but it wouldn't be as complete as it was.

Kirk Caldwell I remember jogging through Waikīkī and it was so eerie. No one. The beach was empty. *And I thought, I'm seeing something I hopefully will never see again in my life.*

David Ige And it happened so quickly. We went from the lowest unemployment rate in the country to the highest in six weeks. Certainly, I was aware that it would impact our economy, but it really shut things down.

With the lockdown and travel quarantine, Hawaiian Airlines, more than ever, was the highway system between the islands, carrying essential workers and cargo.

Peter Ingram (Hawaiian Airlines) Come April 2020, we were flying four round-trip flights—Honolulu to Maui, Līhuʻe, Kona, Hilo—a daily flight to Los Angeles and a daily flight to San Francisco that generated much more revenue from cargo, below the floor, than it did passengers above. But we thought it was important to keep connectivity for both passengers and cargo for essential travel. And of course, for the Neighbor Islands, we were the only game in town. We were carrying healthcare workers, we were carrying electricity repair people—we've always sort of known that that's the highway system of the state, and it was very true when the only people who were traveling were essential workers. It was important to them that we kept the highway system operating.

ESSENTIAL BUSINESS

Banks were considered essential services, but the way of doing business changed dramatically to protect customers and employees alike.

Peter Ho (Bank of Hawaiʻi) Hand sanitizer, wipes, toilet paper, and bottled water—the usual right? Spam and rice too. And we still have a year's supply of PPE. I think we're going to give it out hopefully as Christmas presents this year (2021). So we were kind of feeling good about ourselves because we'd gotten out ahead. We were able to secure all those things and I think now looking back on all of this, the employees, they understood. One of the things I also thought about was hopefully we would all get through this fine—we haven't had any employee fatalities—and then a year from now, or two years from now, you'd be looking back at some point wondering how your employees and customers thought about how you handled the situation. You hope that they'll think you did pretty darn well. Stay focused and keep the plan pretty simple—that's what we tried to do.

Kirk Caldwell Do you think your employees were frightened?

Peter Ho Oh, they were scared. We have 2,100—about a third of them were essential so they had to be on-site and the other two-thirds generally were on-site but we sent them home and they were able to work at home. You had to be focused on this new way of working. And now it seems like second nature—no one wants to come back.

We were so fortunate that, just pure coincidence, we just happened to have spent the last several years modernizing all of that (information technology), so, thankfully, we flipped the switch and all the lights went on like a Christmas tree.

The other issue was the on-site staff, and one of the interesting things that was revealed when we looked back on this story was how much they had to endure. People were frightened, but they had to cash their checks, so they had to come in. Could the money pass along the virus? And it turns out, probably not, but we didn't know a year ago. And you know what? Our people, they didn't flinch. And these people, they're not working for millions of dollars. They're working to pay the rent. Our people were incredible. So that helped fortify us. We had a mission and one of our missions was to live up to our end of the bargain to our staff, which is why we did meals to go and stuff like that.

Kirk Caldwell Did you ever worry that there could be a run on the bank and things would start to fall apart, like in those pandemic movies?

Peter Ho We ordered extra cash in the event that there was a run on cash. Turns out there never was. Never was. I think that's a great testament to the banking industry. People never thought that the system would go down. But we also had lots of redundancies in place around systems. What happens if one of our lockbox teams gets sick? The whole team gets sick? Well you gotta process the lockbox because if you don't process the lockbox Hawaiian Electric doesn't get their money.

So, we had an A team and a B team, and they were never together so we could double our probabilities of not having a real bad problem. Thankfully, we never had to rely on those things. We probably indexed a little bit above the state in terms of rate of infection, which you would expect because we were open for business and we had a younger staff. But we didn't have any deaths and we only found one instance of community spread and it was a really stupid incident and we immediately corrected it. So our managers and leaders were really good in how we dealt with it. We were pretty militant.

Kirk Caldwell You're the president and CEO of a major financial institution in the state of Hawai'i, and the City locks down on a Monday at 4:30. Then the State follows, and the State also announces that no people can come into Hawai'i without quarantining for fourteen days and everything shuts down except for essential businesses. What are you thinking?

Peter Ho What have we done? I just thought, again, it kind of comes down to the math, and maybe if we were in a different business I would have thought a lot differently, but when every day you bring in 30,000 fresh candidates and you're a population of a million four dispersed across a bunch of islands with a great but relatively thin healthcare system, are we really going to take that chance?

Across the street, Bob Harrison at First Hawaiian Bank had also prepared well in advance before the lockdown. First Hawaiian has about two thousand employees throughout Hawai'i, Guam, and Saipan.

Bob Harrison We all got together and talked about it. We have an emergency management system for situations like this. There's a team of people that get together. Turned out that was a good team for a natural disaster, but not the right people for a pandemic. So we made some decisions then on how we're going to respond and how we're going to protect people, as well as how we're going to work through kids not going to school. All of that has downstream impacts on our employees and who could show up for work the next day. The calling trees all got launched;

the managers talking to supervisors who then talk to employees. *Which of you can come to work? How is that going to work?* All of those issues.

We were the first ones to get the plexiglass. We got the last local supply through a customer, and a contractor that did all the work for us said that's not going to be anywhere near enough. So we sourced in Singapore a large load of plexiglass—more than we needed—and we airfreighted it in from Singapore. Luckily, it arrived before all the planes shut down. By then we're already talking about temporarily closing a bunch of branches because nobody's outside. You don't need to have your branch open in Waikīkī when there's nobody in Waikīkī. We had enough plexiglass for the frontline people and then you need to make enough for the people in operations. And then we split our operations center between our main operations center and our disaster recovery site. All these are hundreds of conversations happening in real time.

We did a lot of communications to get the word out. One of the first things we did was talk to Ray Vara from Hawaiʻi Pacific Health, the team at HMSA, and the leadership at Queen's. We also hired an infectious disease expert that could consult with us, and that was in the first couple days. Everyone triangulated on the same person, and he's been phenomenal. He's still working with us, anytime, day or night. He's been a great asset with us, and we want to keep him around forever. You want to have that relationship because you don't know when it's going to happen again.

Fortunately, with so many people being at home then, we didn't have a lot of people who said, "I can't come to work today. I need to take care of my kids or my *kupuna*." We did have people who said, "I'm moving out of"—say, their multigenerational household. "If I'm seeing the public, I can't be around Mom and Dad. They're in their eighties." We tried to advise on that. Everybody was making those decisions. Basically, in that late February to late March time frame, all that got done.

Kirk Caldwell Did you worry at all that there could be a meltdown of our financial system?

Bob Harrison The functioning financial system? I didn't hear from anybody that that was an issue. Exactly what you'd think would have happened by the Fed [Federal Reserve] is what they did. And they're rock stars in this, by the way. Responded very quickly, very strongly, saying it's not a financial issue—it's a health issue. But there's cash everywhere. We were getting extra shipments of cash and they were talking to us very proactively. "Do you have enough? Just let us know. You'll get everything you need." That happened in the first couple days.

Our folks were ordering extra cash. It comes out of the San Francisco Fed even though our contact is at one of the other Federal Reserve Banks, our cash contact. We just wanted to make sure, so we were ordering lots and lots of extra cash. We have a fair amount anyway, but typically in natural disasters people go to cash. That didn't happen this time. But we just brought in a bunch extra just in case. It's the cost of doing business. It sits there and doesn't earn you anything, but that's okay. You need to have that trust, and if someone says I want cash, you give them what they request. And we did have some customers, not too many, but probably a couple hundred people, that wanted to take out cash and put it in the mayonnaise jar, dig a hole in the yard. No, it's not good to have a couple hundred thousand dollars of cash around the house. It's really a bad idea. Most people we were able to talk out of it, but not everybody's going to listen.

Paul Yonamine (Central Pacific Bank) At that point, we were very fortunate at the bank because we had been investing in technology so at least on our internal communication platform we were able to work remotely already. So that part of the lockdown transition was fine. A run on the bank, however, that was a concern. We went ahead and ultimately raised some subordinated debt to add more capital for the bank. None of the other banks did that, but we did that as a safety measure. We raised $56 million in additional monies just in case things turned to the worst. Initially, we didn't get the sense whatsoever from our customers that they were scared. Our branch personnel talked to our customers frequently to reassure them. We also reached out personally to our big customers. And I wasn't even on Zoom—I was constantly making telephone calls to check in with everyone. Everyone was still fine in the beginning so I didn't feel that the bank was in danger at that point, but having said that, I could tell that our customers' operations were going to be significantly impacted over time. In talking with my chief financial officer, we decided to raise the loan loss reserves and get prepared for some challenging times. That was another reason why we raised more capital.

I think the most important thing that we did was to communicate with our employees. I told them early on that they had a safety net. I wasn't going to lay anybody off. At my age, I'll go down with the sinking ship. But I wanted my employees to know that they didn't have to worry about their jobs. They could worry about COVID, but they wouldn't have to worry about their jobs and making ends meet. That was one message that we put out right up front. And then naturally we kicked in with business contingency planning and implemented all the necessary healthcare measures, such as social distancing and guidelines for the branches on PPE. We created a COVID office. We appointed a project manager to it and we executed. As a result, we were somewhat more comfortable because of our level of preparedness.

For rainy days, we continued to raise more capital. We did everything we could to keep everyone healthy. But more importantly, we did what we did so that customers didn't have to worry. And sometimes that was difficult because I would go on a call and have to act the part of being calm despite the fact that I was very nervous. Pre-pandemic, we had just kicked off a forty-million-dollar infrastructure project. And here I was thinking, nobody's coming into the bank now and here we are still spending $40 million. They were interesting calls. But, that's what leadership is all about. Somebody's got to show how to not waste people's time by worrying about things that can't be controlled. That's what my role was all about.

Kirk Caldwell None of us really knew how long this pandemic would last. We still don't know. We thought we were seeing it coming to an end, and now we see more cases than ever. As a banker, how do you manage that, particularly when you are looking for some predictability as you make decisions?

Paul Yonamine By taking it one day at a time. One thing I've accepted is that nobody was an expert on COVID in the beginning. Since the pandemic started, I've learned a lot about the Spanish flu that happened a hundred years ago, and if we had someone who had lived through that experience then that person would have known what to do. But nobody knew about pandemics in 2020, and I certainly had no idea. I strive to be up to date, but even I found so much conflicting information about COVID that it was hard to know what to do. I was reading everything, watching everything, listening to everything, and the advice was all so divided. I took in as much information as I could and then made the best calls that I could. And I had to make the calls for the bank, right or wrong, which I was comfortable doing. I do that all the time: make one decision and then if I have to course correct, I'll correct it. I'm not that proud. I can make mistakes, but I always use my best judgement with the information I have at the time. The one thing I have to admit—and I'll be very open about this—was that I had a lot of frustration with government. I did. Today, though, I look at where we all are and realize that nobody was an expert on this at the time. We were all well intentioned and trying to do the best for ourselves and each other.

The one thing that government could have done better was to assure the people that we would be okay. We would get through this. Unfortunately, there were a lot of people who were running scared and yet the pandemic was totally out of their control. Sometimes there's no reason or explanation to lean on, but leaders still have to be viewed as confident and reassuring. If anything, that's the kind of leadership we could have used a little bit more of.

Sherry Menor-McNamara, CEO of the Chamber of Commerce Hawai'i, had a tough job assisting businesses, being their advocate, and helping them survive amidst a public health crisis.

Sherry Menor-McNamara No one knew how long the pandemic would last, what the rules and regulations were, because at the time they were constantly changing. How do they manage the situation when they're shutting their doors and can't operate? We were simultaneously calling members, finding out if they're okay and what their needs were, coordinating webinars, getting information out on the kinds of PPE that were needed, managing their employees working from home, reconfiguring their office space—whatever was relevant at the moment, we quickly jumped on it. We organized webinars and opened them up to nonmembers to participate as well. At that point, it wasn't about membership. It was about saving the broader business community and ensuring that we were providing what was needed.

Kirk Caldwell Were you able to find resources—whether it be PPE or plexiglass, different types of masks—and share them?

Sherry Menor-McNamara We had businesses reach out to us. For example, AlohaMask.com, Shelley Wilson's company. They said, "We have lots of inventory available at this type of price." Whatever information businesses had available was posted on our COVID resources website.

Paycheck Protection Program (PPP) was a lot more complicated. One, limited funding. Two, you had to go through your financial institution, and not everyone has a bank relationship. Three, how do you fill out the applications? So we had numerous webinars on PPP, these Small Business Administration–backed loans, walking business owners through the application process.

Kirk Caldwell How else did you assist businesses?

Sherry Menor-McNamara We considered ourselves a hub of information. Whatever information we had was disseminated through our communication channels. And, we organized virtual informational events. We also played an advocacy role during that time. As the voice of business in Hawai'i, it was a role that we had to play to elevate the voice of small local businesses because many were at a point of desperation. These businesses had a lot of uncertainties and ran out of resources. A lot of them used personal loans and personal savings, or tried to find different ways to get funding outside of the federal support.

At this point in time, people did not know what was going to happen. We thought we were going to open in a month or two, but it was prolonged.

Kirk Caldwell When O'ahu shut down in the middle of March, how did you find out?

Sherry Menor-McNamara Through the media. So that was another thing. I think business felt that there was no heads up to help them prepare. And there were a lot of questions. *What does a shutdown mean? For how long? What do we do? Does it mean closing operations entirely?* There was the unknown factor that raised a lot of questions. Businesses operate best when there is some level of certainty.

What we heard often was, *Why are we forced to shut down if we're doing everything that we're told to do? We're following all health and safety protocols. We have no cases.* I think they were just questioning, *Why us? We're essential too.* That was another one. *How can they say we're not essential?* There was such an inconsistency. For example, Inspiration Furniture couldn't deliver, but yet Costco and the big box stores could deliver? Local business, especially, felt that they were being punished and weren't being treated on an equal or level playing field.

And then some businesses were seeing other businesses not following the protocols, yet *they* were being forced to shut down? It was an equity issue and a lot of businesses were feeling they are doing the right thing, so why were they being forced to shut down?

A lot of businesses thought they were essential. They saw other businesses operate and said, "If they're essential, then we should be essential." That kind of thing. We got a lot of calls on what is considered an essential business.

So, finally, we said, okay, there's no state programs so let's come up with some ideas: the Hawai'i Restaurant Card program, Hawaii Business Pivot Grant program. The Business Pivot grant program was to ensure that businesses were able to pivot in the current climate. So, fortunately, with the support of the administration and legislative leaders, we received funding for those two programs. The Restaurant Card program helped stabilize the restaurant industry and its supply chain, and the Business Pivot grant helped small and local businesses.

Kirk Caldwell How much of a difference did the Restaurant Card program make?

Sherry Menor-McNamara It was a two to one multiplier, generating more than $150 million on a $75 million program. And, it saved over two thousand jobs.

We had UHERO (University of Hawai'i Economic Research Organization) do an analysis on what kind of impact it would have and then after the program ended we did a final analysis. It provided a $500 gift card to families who lost their jobs to have a nice dinner that normally they could not cover. There was one recipient in Hilo who said, "I have a family, but I don't get to have this kind of food, dining out, treating a family of six for Thanksgiving." Those kinds of stories.

Kirk Caldwell We opened up probably slower than what the Chamber wanted, but faster than what the medical community wanted. By May/June everything was open, including bars. We had some good days of zero cases and then we started seeing increases in cases. Fourth of July was not good. What were you hearing from your members at that point?

Sherry Menor-McNamara As cases were rising consistently, businesses felt, *Oh no, we can't afford this.* There was a fear there would be another shut down and the PPP money was already used.

TRAVEL SHUTDOWN

David Ige (Governor of Hawai'i) Because Hawai'i Tourism Authority (HTA) had the experience with SARS, they were very much concerned. Even though we didn't have SARS cases in the Islands, Japan shut down because they were concerned about travel, they were concerned about SARS being in Hawai'i, and then they all shut everything down.

We knew that the virus was being spread by people traveling, because that was pretty obvious. And our isolation was helpful, but we also knew that our economy was driven by travel.

Kirk Caldwell Did we see a drop off in travel to Hawai'i prior to the government taking action?

David Ige The international travel really wasn't that significantly impacted, even from the continent. The winter is the peak season and we had come off a banner year. We made ten million visitors in 2019. The economic projections were that 2020 was going to be another great year. The budget was based on that, and so certainly we had anticipated that the state was in a strong position, but obviously because of what happened we had to monitor and make sure to be prepared to take action.

Kirk Caldwell So, travel from Asia remained strong until the quarantine?

David Ige Yeah, in fact, we had record numbers year over year by comparison. Spring is the shoulder season and typically we get less travel in February and March, but through the end of March we still had record arrivals year over year. So I think if you compared March 2020 to March 2019, we had more visitors arrive here and so we definitely were concerned about what would happen, and then it became obvious we had to shut things down.

Kirk Caldwell When did you realize this was going to be a defining moment for Hawai'i? That a major crisis was approaching and it would require all hands on deck?

David Ige Certainly in March, as we had to look at a more strict response. There are a couple things. There was so much that we didn't know. We didn't know the nature of the virus, we didn't know how severe the illness would be, there was no vaccine, and there was no treatment. Just because of the uncertainty, we knew that this was going to be a significant challenge—not clear yet that it was going to be the entire planet that would be inundated. It never really happened before.

Previous infectious diseases were typically regional or isolated, so it was not clear that it would expand to cover every place. But I also recognized that Hawai'i would be more vulnerable than elsewhere because the entire visitor economy was built on trying to establish global channels. There's no other destination on the planet that is as connected as Hawai'i is to every place around the world.

Kirk Caldwell Most isolated but the most connected.

David Ige Yeah and that was conscious. It was a specific design that we had because we knew that that would give us the most diverse visitor industry that we could get. I was actively working on bringing Southwest Airlines to the state of Hawai'i, and we finally got them to come in and they had this massive expansion plan, which would have made a tremendous difference. So like I said, we had anticipated that 2020 would be another banner year. Southwest was coming, ANA (All Nippon Airlines) announced their Honu service to Hawai'i and I had gone on a trip to Japan to promote it. I met with the executives at ANA to talk about Hawai'i, wanting them to make Hawai'i their priority destination and they revamped their entire thinking to focus on Japan/Hawai'i. The new Airbus A380s, they had shifted their thinking to make the Hawai'i–Japan route the premier route. So everything was geared toward 2020. Hawai'i was the destination that JTB promoted worldwide. So we had anticipated that Hawai'i 2020 would be a terrific year and as you saw the cases unfold across the country we knew that the coronavirus would definitely have an impact.

The economic impact to Hawaiian Airlines was perhaps the most dramatic.

Peter Ingram People hate uncertainty. And you've got to communicate. There were all sorts of rumors going on, so we ended up having to deploy a whole bunch of different vehicles for getting information out. We had regular emails that go out to people, but not everybody reads email, like those of us who sit at a desk all day. I also recorded videos. Pretty quickly, we started having people in our administrative staff work remotely. We had never used Microsoft Teams before and now I've got Teams wired in this conference room. It's become the go-to application for us, so we rolled that out pretty quickly, even before the stay-at-home orders were part of what we were dealing with.

You can't underestimate the importance of communication because that uncertainty is awful for people. And of course, people are fearful for their health, they're fearful for their livelihood. Ours is a business where not only is your pay for most of our employees based on their seniority, but a lot of things that affect quality of life. Like your bidding schedule and your vacation schedule are based on seniority, so no one wants to see that hierarchy altered. Because as soon as someone leaves off the bottom, you're getting closer to the bottom as opposed to moving towards the top.

So, it was a lot, and we were having to do things to preserve the finances of the business. No revenue was coming in. In fact, cash was going out from tickets because we were doing more refunds than we were booking tickets. For a long period of time, what's normally our revenue inflows were negative numbers. We had more cancellations and refunds than we did new bookings, so we had to do things to reduce our expenses.

Some of that happens naturally, right? If you're not flying, you're not consuming fuel, you're not paying landing fees, but you've still got all the aircraft, rent expenses, fixed costs of this building, you've got computer systems.

Kirk Caldwell What you describe sounds pretty brutal.

Peter Ingram Yeah, there are some parts of the world where rent was forgiven but generally that is in a bankruptcy restructuring situation and we were working very hard not to be in that situation. We did work with a lot of vendors on deferrals in some cases. We worked with vendors on adjusting contract minimums when we weren't using it, but we did not end up renegotiating any of our aircraft leases. We did get some relief when some of the airports we serve, including the airports here in Hawai'i, sort of pushed payments out into the future.

For us, when the CARES Act came along, and the airlines were singled out for federal support from that, one of the conditions was we weren't to lay anyone off until at least the end of October initially, and that got extended with other versions of the Payroll Support Program, which supported airlines.

What we were able to do, and we did do, was if people wanted to voluntarily take time off, then we would do that. So that became one of the things we were communicating, and this was one of the hardest video messages I had to deliver—asking people if they have the means and the desire to take time away from their work. Normally, you want people to be engaged with their work and taking care of our duties, and instead I was delivering very different messages. That was what we had to do to cut costs… and then we had to go and raise a lot of money. And that money raising went on for months, trying to borrow money against aircraft.

Kirk Caldwell You're borrowing this money, but no one knows how long this pandemic is going to last. There is no vaccine on the horizon. No one knows when is it going to be developed, let alone distributed.

Peter Ingram And ultimately we likely have borrowed much more money than we needed. At the time, we were looking at an asymmetric risk, right? If you run out of money, then the business is gone and we're in bankruptcy and there's no recovering. If you borrow too much, you're going to be paying some extra costs, interest costs for a while, and some of that money is going to be locked in long term, but the risk of that versus the risk of financial survival wasn't even a question. We had to go and borrow whatever money we could.

Kirk Caldwell On top of this, you probably had the visitor industry and customers calling every day regarding travel related questions.

Peter Ingram First of all, we had all sorts of customers calling because they wanted to adjust their travel plans. They had bookings. People could have either credits, or if we canceled flights we had refunds, but we couldn't handle all the calls. We were overrun in our reservations center. We actually spooled up a reservation center here on this floor—the floor where the corporate offices are located—and trained people to have some of the skills to be able to just process cancellations, which were what most of those calls were about. We knew why people were calling, so we just trained people to do that one thing.

But you're right. There was a lot of contact at different levels of government. Ours is a federally regulated business. We spend time with the State on certain labor matters and with the airport, and we spend time with the Counties on certain matters, but by and large we're federally regulated. Well, once we had that quarantine in place, we were state regulated too. So I spent a lot of time—and Ann Botticelli spent a lot of time—with government relations, so there was that level of communication.

Kirk Caldwell You must have been working seven days a week and sixteen to twenty hours a day through March/April?

Peter Ingram It was pretty busy. And through the time that the CARES Act was passed, there was a lot of coordination with our A4A board, which is all the CEOs for the US airlines and of course they're all headquartered mostly in eastern and central time zones. Alaska's on the west coast, we're out here, the trade association is in Washington, DC, so all those meetings were generally oriented around East Coast time zones. So, it was sort of 3:30 in the morning conference calls that we'd start there and then you'd be on Hawai'i time for other meetings, so it was pretty hectic there for a while.

THE MEDICAL COMMUNITY RESPONSE

The decision to lock down was greatly influenced by the impact of the virus on the state's health system and hospital capacity.

Libby Char (Hawai'i DOH) A lot of us in the medical community had been clamoring for a shutdown before it came. *What are we waiting for?* We knew the longer we waited the more cases we would have. Once it was seeded, it was going to be really difficult if not impossible to get rid of. And the feeling was that we have this wonderful border called the Pacific Ocean and we should take advantage of it. I think a lot of the medical community didn't understand that you cannot prevent airplanes from coming in, that there are federal regulations and laws—it's not that easy. But just from a medical standpoint, people were clamoring, *Shut it down, shut it down.*

The medical community by and large was hoping somebody would make a decision and shut it down long before that happened. I shouldn't speak on behalf of the entire medical community, but that was my sense. At least the people I had been talking to. *What are they waiting for? Shut it down. Take advantage of our borders. Shut it down.*

Kirk Caldwell We announced the O'ahu lockdown on Sunday, and on Monday at 4:30 it took effect. What were you starting to see as we went into this?

Libby Char In some ways it was a sigh of relief that somebody had taken action. And that it got everybody and the public out of the confusion we were dealing with. First responders and the people in the healthcare system still had to go to work and deal with this. So it kind of removed all of that uncertainty and I think the good thing is that it allowed healthcare and first responders and all those who were on the front line having contact with COVID patients to then seriously ramp up planning, preparation, and implementation. It removed a lot of extraneous noise to allow those that needed to really start solidifying plans to do so. And so, in some ways it was a relief and it was a really big wake-up call. We're in it now. The bell has been rung. All hands on deck. It was a very interesting paradox because everything that was shut down became very quiet. And at the same time on the healthcare side, it really became very noisy.

Kirk Caldwell I like the way you describe it. It became quiet on the outside, in our community, but a lot of noise on the inside, on the healthcare side of it. You folks were getting ready.

Libby Char We had escaped MERS-CoV, the Middle East respiratory virus that had killed thousands of people—we had escaped that in Hawai'i. We really, for the most part, had escaped Ebola. We had done preparations for it, but we didn't have patients here calling 911. We had escaped SARS, and even H1N1 didn't affect a lot of people here. These were all things that happened in other places, but not here. All of a sudden it really was here and it was kind of like, *Oh (expletive), what do we do?* At the time, there was only limited knowledge and understanding about this virus and there was no treatment.

We didn't know whether our plans really would work. They were about to be tested in a huge way. At the time, we didn't realize that. How could we realize it? So for us, this really was our first foray into actually responding, unlike the rest of the world that had already dealt with some of the other infectious diseases.

Ray Vara (Hawai'i Pacific Health) Fortunately, at HPH, we've got a leadership team that's been together for a long time. Melinda Ashton, Art Gladstone, Martha Smith—all these leaders who have worked together literally for almost two decades. We were all working out of our command center along with the rest of the management team.

Jonathan Dworkin (Queen's Health System) I think the lockdown order that you guys did was probably the first big effective thing in terms of reducing transmission. And I don't think it was too late because what we saw in the hospital (Queen's) was that that first wave that peaked at the beginning of April was something like twenty-five, thirty admissions, maybe twenty admissions in the hospital, which was much smaller than the later waves. So it succeeded in blunting that first wave. And it was just in time. I think if you had waited another week or two we would have been looking at a much bigger mortality event.

But if you look at the chronology, if you compare Hawai'i to New York, De Blasio and Cuomo, it doesn't look good for those guys. They basically waited until they had thousands of circulating cases. And then when they shut down, they had a mass mortality event.

Kirk Caldwell It's good to know we did it just in time. If the DOH had been more proactive earlier, we probably would have taken action earlier and been able to better manage the caseload going forward. We'll get into the testing, tracing, and isolation issues, which we pushed hard early on and were shut down by the DOH. To this day I don't understand why DOH was so slow in reacting to the impending pandemic crisis.

How serious a problem did you think this was going to be? Did you think it was going to be a major health event not only for our state but also for our country?

Jonathan Dworkin Around the same time, I was looking at the case fatality rate and also some of the social and economic indicators around it. What was happening with mobility? What was happening with air travel? What was happening with border control? What was happening in cities with things like restaurant pedestrian traffic and business? And what you saw in every place where there was an explosion of cases was just a complete shutdown. A complete lockdown. And it's not that that happened because people were so keen to do that—in most places people didn't want to do those things. But what happened was the hospitals started filling up and when the hospitals started filling up people realized they had a crisis on hand and that the hospital wasn't going to work, and then you had to shut everything down.

Even in places where there was resistance to those types of measures, like in Bergamo in Northern Italy, where the business community basically ran that province and had done everything they could to minimize the threat of COVID, they still ended up going under lockdown. And a very prolonged lockdown.

So I noticed that and I thought, *When it gets here we're going to be paralyzed by it. We're going to be shut down. And whether we want to be or not, the only thing you have control over is how many people end up dead. One way or another, it's going to shut us down.*

I wasn't under any illusion that it was as deadly as smallpox or something like that. The fatality rate was never that high. Never 30 percent or 50 percent. I think I saw it as more of a threat because of its contagiousness and its ability to spread and its ability to overwhelm healthcare systems and then shut down normal life. And then the question was *How can we continue with enough normal life so that we can get through this without having people go hungry and whatnot?* Those were the types of things on my mind and when I wrote the leap day post, I tried to warn people about this. I said it's not going to be that everyone's dying on the street 'cause it's not that deadly of an infection, but it's not going to be normal life either. Things are going to be weird, different, and nothing in our lifetimes can prepare us for what it's like to be in Bergamo, Italy, during a pandemic, where you see entire towns under lockdown. I thought that that was likely. And then we would have to figure out how to navigate through it going forward until we had a better treatment.

Kirk Caldwell So, you're at Queen's and you're making your views known. What about outside of Queen's? You're watching our State, our City, government leaders, business leaders, and we ended up reaching out to you. Hiro Toiya, the director of the Department of Emergency Management (DEM), is a hero for finding you, but I wish we would have found you earlier.

Jonathan Dworkin You guys created a monster when you brought me in. The early thing I wanted to set up in addition to testing was quarantine. I thought, *Visitor numbers are dropping off now. We've got all these empty hotel rooms. We've got to set up some kind of centralized quarantine so that we can keep those people who are sick separate from those who are not sick. We don't have testing, we don't have isolation, we don't have contact tracing, we don't have centralized quarantine, we don't have any of the public health planks we need to succeed in the pandemic.*

And one of the things I started doing was making a lot of noise because I couldn't discharge COVID patients safely because the State had never set up quarantine. There was no place to discharge them. A lot of these people were coming from crowded housing, and I was making a big fuss. A lot of my colleagues were saying, "Why are you making so much noise?" What's the expression? The squeaky tire gets the grease?

Kirk Caldwell The squeaky wheel gets the oil.

Jonathan Dworkin I was calling the Queen's administration saying, "I can't safely discharge these people because HI-EMA hasn't set up the damn hotel. Are you guys going to set up the hotel?" So, Queen's admin starts trying to get hotel rooms. I think that was the City's entry point around that time. Hiro Toiya was helping with those things. And the next thing I know, Hiro is inviting me to meet you. So that's where your path and my path, I think, intersect.

David Derauf (Kōkua Kalihi Valley) I think our community was supportive of the lockdown. People felt it was for the right thing. We didn't really see any resistance. What we did see, however, in the Pacific Island community, particularly the Micronesian community, was that there was not much outreach to them. They rely on their own channels of communication, including social media in their own language. There wasn't much public health messaging and, as you can recall, it was already very political. So if you were associated with a church that was very conservative, you might be getting your message from President Trump, saying, "Ah, we don't need masks." So, I think that was a problem in our community.

The second and most important thing is we knew from the get-go that given how crowded the housing is here in our community, we couldn't quickly get people out of the house if they were infected. You're going to see everyone in that household becoming infected. My personal record is twenty-one people in a one-bedroom apartment. That's in terms of crowdedness. And I thought, *Twenty-one people with a respiratory virus. That's twenty-one cases. That's twenty-one cases that are going to be four hundred cases, and that was borne out.*

As we saw last summer at this time (2020), a large percentage of the cases were coming out of this community, Kalihi, especially public housing.

Kaua'i mayor Derek Kawakami at the beginning of the lockdown also ordered a nighttime curfew for the island, and he understood that it was a hardship for families. As a personal response, he created videos on social media for his community to provide information and entertainment and also to show that he and his family were abiding by the same restrictions.

Derek Kawakami I'm a weirdo. That's who I am. The island elected somebody that's more comfortable out at the base yards with the guys wearing the hard hats and the blaze orange shirts than I am with the other executives and leaders. That's where I feel I'm a fish out of water. I play softball, I surf, I hunt, I love shooting guns—I'm just an average joe that got lucky. That's the kind of stuff we do as a family. We open windows for people to peek into our personal life because my wife was a schoolteacher for about eighteen, nineteen years.

Demographically, where you have a high percentage of low- to moderate-income families, the first thing she said as we were keeping kids at home was that for some of these kids their only meal was when they come to school. She would see all these things. She's on the front line with the good, the bad, and the ugly of society. The only time they're not getting yelled at by their parents is when they're in school. She knew that this whole stressful situation was just going to intensify all the bad in our community.

So she said there's got to be a way we can feel like the kids. The primary thing was my wife and daughter said let's try to do something where we can at least provide some joy for the kids. That was just when we did the curfew. And she said we have to also let our people know that we're under the same rules as everybody else, that we're at home every night, we're all in this curfew together. We gotta do it every night. I said, "Oh my god. We'll do a few." The first night we did board games. The second night we did baking. And the third night, I said, "We're going to teach our people how to take care of themselves. We're going to teach them how to make masks."

Geez, but we did one every single night. And a lot of people appreciated it, us reaching out, but at the same time social media became like a toxic environment for my wife, my family, myself, and I said, "Eh, when we lift this curfew, we're going to take a break from social media because it's not adding value and positivity to our personal life. Right now people can turn real negative, and I don't want to expose my daughter to this nonsense." We kind of took a big break from social media. I don't think people realize how much work goes into one of those crafts demonstrations and this became really tedious. I would come home, and Monica and Haley would be waiting there because they were teaching and learning from home, spending all this time at home, and I was like, *My god, couldn't we have chosen something a little easier to do?* Because it became like an hour and a half, two hours just trying to pull these things off and get it out to people in time. If we were twenty minutes late, they were like, "Where's the next episode?" Holy mackerel.

But it was fun for me, for our family. It was fun for my wife and daughter. It was fulfilling for me to know that we were helping people get through very stressful times. At least for a brief moment in time, we were taking their mind off of COVID-19.

Kirk Caldwell to David Ige Was the shutdown your most difficult decision?

David Ige (Governor of Hawai'i) I think that it was. We're impacting everything, every activity, asking people because of this virus to stay at home and I know that the state wasn't equipped for people to work at home. So I think those were the two things that were most difficult, the stay-at-home order and the quarantine, because clearly it would touch everything that happened in the state.

The support, generally, from the community was very strong. They followed and complied with restrictions, and many businesses were willing to support the decision. I think it still comes back to the fact that we're an island community and I know it's the cliché about aloha spirit, but I think everyone here is prepared to sacrifice on behalf of the community. And they would have done it over and over and over again. The public response to an emergency is always overwhelming. Everybody without even asking is willing to sacrifice to help others. It was heartwarming to see the public response. Yes, it was a difficult decision. We knew that it would impact virtually everybody and every organization in the state of Hawai'i, but I also felt confident that people would respond as they have in the past. That people understood that there is a broader purpose and that they are willing to sacrifice individual conveniences on behalf of the community in general.

My naive and optimistic perspective was that it would be a short period of time, and that we would get to a better place, then we would be able to get on with our lives, even though we didn't know much at that time.

Just a couple things about that shutdown. Part of that is when you look at exempting all essential businesses, essentially the only businesses that get shut down are the small family businesses. It's easy for the big guys to say, "Yeah, shut everything down." And by the way, banks and financial institutions are already essential businesses, and I'm not going to shut them down. Grocery stores are essential businesses. So really when you say we're shutting everything down, well not really. You're just shutting down the small guys. So the question that I had at that point is *Is there another way to try to slow the spread of the virus without having to shut down the small businesses?* And then you heard the same criticisms I've heard from the small businesses: "Look, there's more people in Costco and Walmart that would ever come into my shop. And those guys are able to operate and you're shutting me down?" ✻

CHAPTER 3

Health vs. Business

In early 2020, an article by Tomas Pueyo entitled "The Hammer and the Dance" aptly described the rhythm of the pandemic. The lockdowns were the hammer, and the quest to reopen involved a delicate dance of saving lives and saving businesses. Hawai'i leaders struggled to learn the steps, cautiously stepping forward, sometimes needing to step back.

Mike Victorino (Mayor of Maui County) After Maui County shut down and started to reopen, I took a systematic and methodical approach. We allowed certain groupings at certain times to see if there were any major outbreaks or impacts because of that particular reopening. After each two- to three-week period, we'd consider opening something else if it was possible. For example, we opened parks and then we started to open gyms, not the public gyms but the private gyms. When the private gyms started to show higher numbers because transmission was occurring in an enclosed environment, we decided to shut them down again.

It was the same with restaurants and bars. When we reopened, we went to ten o'clock with no dancing or karaoke allowed. We tried to make it so that if there was a particular outbreak we could pinpoint the cause and either shut it down and/or try to minimize the impact of that outbreak situation.

Georgette Deemer How did the business community do? Did you have a lot of businesses and restaurants that had to shut forever?

Mike Victorino Sadly, yes, we had some. In every county there were businesses that either couldn't survive or, for them, returning to full operations just didn't make good sense. For some mom-and-pop operations, the owners said, "Enough." Some had been thinking about retirement and closing down anyway, and the pandemic was a good reason at that point to say, "Okay, we're retiring." While for some, it was more of a timing issue. So, some operations will never return.

But most of our restaurants and bars have returned (this was as of summer 2021). I would say a good 65 percent have opened back up and, with the large number of visitors on Maui now, they're doing quite well, except they can't find enough help. That's the challenge we face. Like on O'ahu and, in fact, throughout the entire nation—people aren't coming back to work. Either they don't feel safe or they're living more comfortably than they did prior to the pandemic.

Georgette Deemer You know, I wanted to let you know that I just finished watching *The White Lotus* (HBO). I know that there's criticism, but I really liked it. They must have shot that in the midst of 2020.

Kirk Caldwell I remember you talking about this, Mayor. You said you were going to support the film industry during the pandemic, when there were very few visitors on Maui, as a way to create economic stimulus for your residents.

Mike Victorino There were two major film projects on Maui that were controversial during what I called the "pre-height" of the pandemic. *Temptation Island* was filmed at the Andaz Maui at Wailea Resort and *White Lotus* was filmed at the Four Seasons, also in Wailea.

Temptation Island was the first one. I caught a lot of backlash from that one. However, we sat down and developed all the safety protocols. Every cast member, every worker was tested each and every day. I believe they did something like nine thousand tests in that three-and-a-half-month period. Bottom line is that not one positive case was reported during filming of *Temptation Island*.

Kirk Caldwell So you did nine thousand tests just for *Temptation*

Island? That's a lot of tests and not one case.

Mike Victorino Not one case was reported. They worked in bubbles. They had certain badges that allowed people only in certain areas. They weren't allowed to get together. There were a lot of protocols we put in place between our medical people and their medical people, and it worked out really well.

When *White Lotus* came along, we followed basically the same procedures. In fact, my wife and I went down to *White Lotus* to watch some of the filming, and we had to get tested before we went and then again when we arrived. And so, for me personally, I've been tested eighteen times already. Almost every month I get tested somehow, somewhere, because of the protocols that are in place.

Kirk Caldwell I've not seen *Temptation Island*, but I saw three episodes of *The White Lotus* and you would never know there's a pandemic. No one's wearing masks, the hotel looks filled. It's amazing how you pulled that off. They must have left a lot of money on your shores in a time when there was very little money coming into Maui.

Mike Victorino I think *White Lotus* brought us almost $60 million in revenue and brought people back to work. That really helped because the production brought back some of the hotel employees to take care of not only the cast, but the people behind the cameras and the support crews. The timing was good. We really needed some help.

Derek Kawakami (Mayor of Kaua'i County) At that time, we were an anomaly. That's when we started Safe Travels, and everybody's cases were coming in, and the scientific evidence was pointing to that a lot of it was community acquired or the people who were taking the pretravel test were coming in negative. But our positives started to go up when we opened up under the State's Safe Travels program. Kaua'i was the complete opposite. Once again, Kaua'i is the black sheep, even when we don't want to be.

The scientific evidence showed that a large number of our cases coming in at that time were people who were taking that pretravel test, arriving on Kaua'i, and then becoming sick and then seeding COVID-19 into the community. So we said, "Look, we're opting out." And people were so mad at us. If you want to know what pressure is from all around, it was there. And that's quite all right because people will realize that I'll deal with the pressure, and our team is built for pressure, so we just held the line. We believed in what we believed in and we weren't looking for consensus. We were looking to give everybody an opportunity to voice their opinion and we learned a lot and incorporated a lot of those opinions. But when you're trying to lead, if you're looking for consensus, you'll never get there.

So we believed in the bubble program, but we knew that was just a stopgap measure. The big problem is, you remember right around that time, the governor really started taking away a lot of the powers that the mayors had prior to that. And it became difficult. He sat on that rule—gosh, it felt like for months. My sense of time is blurred because this thing has gone on so long, but it seemed like a long time that they sat on it and then, finally said, "Go, give it a go."

We knew our island; we're not O'ahu. I told the governor, "Look, 30 percent of inventory of our rooms are actually hotels. Another 30 percent are time-shares. So these are people who are going to stay for about two weeks. So being in a resort bubble for a few days is not an issue because they bought the time-share prior to coming. And the other market, 20 percent or so, are vacation rentals. So their average length of stay is longer. We have a market in place, so let's give it a go, give it a try. My god, how many opportunities do we have to see if these things work?"

If we have another pandemic, you're going to have to put something in place and a proof of concept, so at least we knew that we could still have at least some of the gears of the economy turning while keeping the island safe. I'm glad the governor eventually gave us a go. The hotels that did participate did okay. They wanted to continue the program and then eventually we just didn't need that model anymore. And hopefully we'll never need it again.

Kirk Caldwell We saw it work and I do think it's a valuable model for the future. And you proved it yourself. I think Timbers Kaua'i [Ocean Club & Residences] was one of them, right?

Derek Kawakami Timbers was one of them. But we did a lot of wacky stuff in the beginning. Besides the curfew, I said we gotta make Kaua'i appealing. We're trying to slow down travel. We had the Hawai'i State Department of Transportation (DOT)—we're telling them, "Don't let the cruise ship guys come in. Let them dock, resupply, but right now our people are going to freak out if they see a whole bunch of guys debarking the cruise ships." And that's when DOT was being, "Oh we don't have the jurisdiction." I was like, "No, you guys have jurisdiction over the harbor. That's owned by the State."

So we did things like, okay, we're gonna do beach park permit fees for nonresidents. I remember like, "How much do you wanna charge, Mayor?" "Thousand bucks!" They were like, "No, you can't charge a thousand bucks. There's got to be a nexus." But we did all of these. When DOT said, "You don't have jurisdiction over harbors—it's the Coast Guard," I would disagree. We were already formulating plans to be like, okay, well, it's a county road that leads to your harbors, so we were ready to, by all means necessary, to protect our vulnerable.

We didn't have anything for our elderly population. We didn't have anything for those with underlying health conditions. And I said, "Eh, we're still a state that keeps our elders as living treasures. We don't just put 'em out to the pasture." Leaders go back to the elders and ask them for advice. We still honor and respect our elders, and for those with underlying health conditions, I said, "Look, our Native Hawaiian population has high levels of high blood pressure, diabetes, heart disease, and my gosh, if we're not going to protect the host culture of our people. So by all means, if necessary, we're gonna take some hits to protect our people." So we took some hits.

Kirk Caldwell I think you're a leader people were looking for. Maybe people are upset about the economy, but everyone trusts you, and there's no one that doesn't think you didn't put their health and safety first.

Derek Kawakami Oh there are tons of people that do not trust me. And there are tons of people that think that, well, there's just different priorities. And I can understand that because I came from the private sector with our own business, Big Save—that's a nickel-and-dime profit margin business. And I can remember one of the first things that I had to do coming back home was to inform associates that we're closing down our gift shop branch. And so what we're doing is we're putting people who never had to get on financial assistance on financial assistance. These were people who had always accepted the responsibility of controlling their own destiny and the destiny of their workers, and all of a sudden there is a loss of that sense of the ability to control their destiny and putting people in the awkward position of having to have their hand out for help. And a lot of people don't know how to do that.

I gotta work hard at making them whole. A lot of people have come around and have seen the bigger picture, but this current situation has them on pins and needles and I just gotta constantly reassure them that we're going to move forward and we're going to be pragmatic and we're going to be very mindful of the consequences that come with our mitigative efforts.

According to Chris Benjamin, for Alexander & Baldwin, the health of the corporation depended on the health and survival of the business tenants across the state.

Chris Benjamin I didn't know how long the pandemic was going to last, I didn't know how many tenants would survive, I didn't know if we would survive. We borrowed $120 million on our revolver within a week or two after this whole thing started to blow up because we thought it was an existential event for us and we knew we were going to have to support our tenants, so we knew we needed cash and we didn't know how much. Fortunately, we paid all that back and it's all fine, but my mantra from day one was it's going to be better to have tenants on the other side of this pandemic than it is to try to backfill a bunch of empty spaces.

So both from a community perspective and humanitarian perspective, but also from a business perspective, it was the right thing to do to be accommodating of our tenants. Now that doesn't mean that we sent everybody a letter and said, "Hey you don't have to pay rent for six months." We worked with each individual tenant.

Some people's businesses took off. Grocery stores did well. There were other tenants who did very well from day one. Other tenants struggled when it was a complete lockdown but then as soon as they figured out a curbside pickup model or they figured out a delivery model or the stores reopened they did better. Other tenants struggled mightily until the tourists came back and now their business is off the chart. Every situation was a little different and we had to tailor our relief to the different situations. I'm sure that not every tenant is thrilled with what we did, but what we tried to do was really focus on their true needs and meet those needs where we could.

Peter Ho (Bank of Hawai'i) I did worry a lot about how long we could hold our breath. And thankfully, we've never seen a fiscal response like we had and people complain about we're putting too much money out in the streets. Well, probably. We probably overdid it, but with the federal system, and as a result, the state and local municipalities, who's to tell what's the right number? And if you're going to do it, you'd be really stupid not to overdo it. And really foolish to underdo it. So if you're gonna do it, you gotta do it. And we'll deal with the consequences later.

Kirk Caldwell I think putting a lot of money into the system helps ensure a return to a stronger economy. Maybe we get some inflation, but you'd much rather have that than have to live through a recession that goes on for five years. And yeah, maybe money was wasted in certain areas, but you also have all this additional growth that you would not have had.

Peter Ho And people will forget very quickly that had we not done that, had the federal government not done that—I was very concerned about anarchy, the system breaking down, which you don't have to be very imaginative to see how that could have happened.

Kirk Caldwell What we appreciated is that you did not give up working with us even though I'm sure it was extremely frustrating and difficult to interface with both the state and county governments at the same time. We're not as nimble as you guys, but you didn't say, "Forget it. I'm going back to my silo." Why did you continue to work with us?

Peter Ho Because we needed to make decisions. Certainly, there was frustration but I think we understood the position that the state, the city and the other counties and other public systems were saddled with. Because, look, nobody is willing to spend the money and resources to outfit a federal, state, and local infrastructure that can perform well in a hundred-year pandemic. It doesn't happen. But then you have a hundred-year pandemic and you got to do the best you can do. So to me it was my responsibility as someone who has a leadership role in the community to try to be supportive. And part of, in my view, in being supportive was to say, hey, here's how I think we should be thinking about this, this is my view, and ultimately you, Mayor, decide and the governor decides, but I'm not just going to fall into line with whatever you say we should do. I'm going to tell you what I think we should do.

Generally, I think businesspeople have the benefit of a profitability behind them and governments do not. Governments, no one gives them an extra helping of dessert if they're right, if they succeed. But if you fail, boy there's a steep price to pay there. I don't know if that's how I'd mention it, but I was sympathetic to it.

As businesses suffered revenue loss during the lockdown, the local banks started to process Paycheck Protection Program loans at an unprecedented rate.

Paul Yonamine (Central Pacific Bank) Our bank originated over eleven thousand loans. Last year (2020), in the first round, there was this limited pot of money, so we were in panic mode, making sure we brought as much money into Hawai'i as we could. Central Pacific Bank underwrote the most Paycheck Protection Program (PPP) loans in Hawai'i and we were working 24/7. My wife was baking cookies for employees past midnight. As it turns out, we made a lot in fee income from the PPP but we didn't think about that as an incentive. Tourists weren't coming and our home was going to tank unless we brought in as much money as we could. So we stepped up and did that. For example, our restaurant clients were dying, so we started Keep Hawaii Cooking and spent a chunk of money subsidizing meals. I think that work reinvigorated the takeout and delivery business here.

We also planted the seeds around Movers and Shakas to bring temporary residents here and that went viral. Another initiative was to help Wahiawa General build out their COVID facility.

But the beauty of all of this was, it wasn't just our bank. For every bank and every company here, it's always about this community. Everyone always gives back to the community. We here in Hawai'i do that much more than any other city or county or state that I know of. I know we do that a lot more than in Japan where I have spent most of my career. I was really proud of that community effort because the community really came together.

Kirk Caldwell Regarding the PPP loans, I was told that Central Pacific Bank did more of these types of loans than it did in the entire year for small business loans.

Paul Yonamine Well, 11,400 loans in round one and two combined. That's a lot of loans. Initially, issuing PPP loans was the most frustrating process because the Small Business Administration portal was so poor. It would freeze then bounce back. Then sometimes it would take two hours just to upload an application, which was frustrating. But the process progressively got better and then finally my digital team in Boulder, Colorado, automated it. And so towards the end of the first round and then into the second round, the PPP loans were a breeze. We had technology that worked, which we offered to a number of other banks. We also sent a group of employees to one bank to teach them our process and were able to offer them the technology as well.

As a result of the PPP loan program, even though our intention was to bring in the money to help Hawai'i, the end result was that we benefitted from the fee income we were getting out of it. A lot of companies also decided to move their accounts to us, so we've actually increased our market share by four points. It's very difficult to do that in Hawai'i. Both outcomes were totally unexpected, as we never intended the PPP loans to work to our advantage.

Personally, I've been really involved with our customers by trying to help them come up with ideas for either cutting costs or increasing their top line, especially around e-commerce and especially the Japan-facing customers. If I had to go through this experience again, I would have tried to help more companies to survive. The economy is roaring back and when the Japanese start returning, we're going to be pretty strong here. Already hotels and most restaurants are going to probably beat the profitability of 2019. But there was this hiccup period in 2020 when a lot of companies went out of business. If I were to do it all over again, I would have helped more companies weather that period.

Bob Harrison (First Hawaiian Bank) We had customers that had four hundred to five hundred employees. I can think of one in particular. A resort retail company here and in the Mainland. They went from 350 employees to five because there was literally no one here and no one in their other resort areas on the Mainland. So then we took 10 percent of our employees, about two hundred people, and they all started doing PPP loans, which was a madhouse.

We were the number one Small Business Administration lender for our size bank three out of the last four years, about fifty to fifty-five loans per year. And we did, in this process, ten thousand PPP loans. So that's the difference. In the first round we did just under six thousand in literally six weeks. Some of our people were coming in, saying, "I quit." They were just so stressed out. All of that's going on at the same time.

Dr. Libby Char described the medical community side of the health vs. business balance.

Libby Char (Hawai'i DOH) I think a lot of friction arose because background and perspective doesn't lend itself to seeing things from the other side so well. The public health issues were pretty straightforward.

This is what we should do for the good of public health. But I think the business community was seeing the economic side of it and obviously the toll it would take on businesses and the economy, and so they wanted to do something else. And I think people had the sense that there were two opposing forces that were fighting each other when in fact they were so joined at the hip.

The challenge for you, Mayor, as the leader is that you had to make the ultimate decision. And so you have two seemingly competing interests knocking on your door, and that's where I think public health has always been in the shadows or had a back seat. Obviously, the business and economic engines have always been involved in politics. That's where a lot of money comes from. They're very influential and they have already established relationships. When public health is functioning as it should, it often is in the background of people's lives and is taken for granted. Public health usually isn't as visible or appreciated in government and I think that is very unfortunate and it created some frustration.

Kirk Caldwell I agree with you about public health being in the back seat. I told Hiro Toiya (director of the DEM) we needed advice from the medical and public health community because at that point the DOH wasn't working very well for the City and County of Honolulu. There was not a strong relationship with the medical community because public health responsibilities fell more to the State of Hawai'i and its health department. The counties do not have health departments.

Libby Char There's no relationship. There's no big money. Your campaign coffers are not going to get replenished on what the public health folks can donate. You are going to do a lot better with the donations coming from the business sector and all your corporate friends. Money talks. It's important that you have business relationships with them. That was a challenge for the public health voice.

It was also challenging to get the public health and medical community to realize that there are other factors that weigh into the decision, not just the medical side. And then to get the business community to understand *We're not your enemy. We're trying to keep the community healthy!* I think some of the business community saw the public health and medical community as being an opponent. That was really frustrating and that was a big problem because from the public health standpoint it was pretty obvious that without a healthy population you weren't going to have a healthy workforce or a healthy economy.

Kirk Caldwell We talked to Peter Ingram at Hawaiian Airlines and he said, way before we took any action, in January, flights coming to Hawai'i from Inchon, South Korea, were becoming more and more empty. Planes coming out of Sapporo, Japan, were more and more empty. That Hawaiian had to cancel flights because people weren't showing up. If we took no action and we had thousands of cases and hospitals were filled, we probably would have had the same lockdown effect but with a lot more sick people.

Libby Char I think that there's a tremendous economic advantage to a county or to the state of Hawai'i being disease-free or having very low rates of disease. That's powerful. And you could attract the kind of visitors you wanted that would have been very responsible just because of that. So if you said, "You can come to our state. It may be expensive and you're going to have to quarantine in these resorts for a week or a couple of weeks," but knowing it was a very safe disease-free or low disease environment, I think that would have been a huge draw for certain visitors.

Kirk Caldwell It's like a statewide bubble. Just like we talked about these bubble hotels.

Libby Char And it has been borne out when you look at the travelers coming here now. We have a lot of people traveling here because they know it's safe here. They know that we can be outdoors, we can go hiking, there are lots of activities, we can go to the beach, we can do the things that people want to do, and it's a pretty safe place to be. There was reluctance on the part of the business and economic community to hold off a little bit longer and ensure that we kept the disease burden down.

And the argument that we're hearing even now to this day is we have capacity in the hospitals and in the ICUs, so we can accept more risk; it's okay if our numbers grow, we've got plenty of capacity in the hospital. (Remember, this was pre-Delta variant and we didn't have many therapeutics or even vaccines early on.) There was no recognition that people would die unnecessarily or end up with long-term effects of COVID infection. I find that really mind-boggling. That that's the thought process that some people have. I think the extent to which we keep our population safe and we keep Hawai'i safe will pay off and I think we're already seeing it with the rebound in the economy being significantly faster than what was predicted. The number of travelers arriving is over thirty thousand a day.

John De Fries (President and CEO, Hawai'i Tourism Authority) My orientation—long before I came to the Hawai'i Tourism Authority (HTA), from the time I started in the industry in 1973 as a tour director—I for one have never seen the community and the industry as two separate entities. And I've often cautioned my colleagues in the industry to avoid talking about the community as if it's a third-person entity somewhat separate from the industry itself. The reality is, 24/7, the community clocks into our various business enterprises, and as a community, we make the visitor industry operational. This relationship between our community and the visitor industry is symbiotic.

Looking back at the summer and fall of 2020 when visitor arrivals plummeted to near zero, it felt euphoric for us as *kama'āina* to see the beaches and parks empty and no traffic congestion. I remember standing in the middle of Kalākaua Avenue one evening, and I couldn't see a moving vehicle in either direction, and it looked like a giant pedestrian mall or a film set.

Kirk Caldwell That's an eerie thing, isn't it? I went to Waikīkī Beach one late afternoon. I jogged around Diamond Head down into Waikīkī and looked at the beach. There was not a person on the beach. I thought, *I'm seeing something that we will never see again in Hawai'i's history.* It was chicken skin.

John De Fries Yeah, very eerie. At that time there were no barricades on the street, so the actual landscape itself was the same, it just didn't have people in it. As kamaʻāina, it felt like we got our space back, our beach back, our island back, but those of us in business and community leadership know that this is not a sustainable scenario. You could sense that a lot of people and families were trapped under this economic collapse. In my mind, it's kind of like going to Ala Moana Center and the second, third, fourth, fifth floor just collapses, and you know you've got people underneath that are trapped—children, kūpuna, all the things you had to worry about as mayor that you know are at risk or being harmed by this economic collapse.

Granted, state and federal subsidies helped to cushion the adverse impacts, but this type of financial support was not going to be a permanent solution. For HTA and our stakeholder partners, the unified focus was to get our visitor industry reopened and on a sustained trajectory toward economic recovery. However, right now in Hawaiʻi, as we are approaching September 2021 and our recovery efforts are still uneven, we're still not on a sustained trajectory. There were good indicators for our recovery up until April and May, but then this Delta variant dealt us a major setback and we're teetering on history repeating itself from a year ago.

At Hawaiian Airlines, we asked Peter Ingram how the 2020 pandemic compared to his experiences in the airline industry after 9/11. Were there lessons learned about helping businesses to recover after a catastrophic disaster?

Peter Ingram September 11th was a different point in my career. I was at American Airlines. I was a managing director in airport customer services. It was an intense period of time, but I wasn't in the seat where every eyeball in the company is on you and what you're doing. Initially, I hated the comparisons to that, having been through 9/11, because that was such a traumatic experience for any airline person to see our assets of good being used as a weapon by people intent on doing evil things. Any comparison to that was hard.

But in terms of the impact on the business, it's not even close. This pandemic was more destructive. We've had far more people who are actual casualties of this in terms of loss of life than we did after 9/11. We were shut down for four days completely as an industry after 9/11 in the US and then traffic recovered over a six-month period. It was pretty quickly—within a couple of months—back to 20 percent below. Well, we didn't get to 20 percent below on Hawai'i traffic until almost a year after the onset of the pandemic crisis. So from an economic impact, this has been far more severe.

Because we didn't know how the disease was spreading initially, we had all sorts of policy decisions where you're trying to follow CDC guidance and we're enhancing the cleaning of the aircraft, we're changing procedures overnight—that was reminiscent of how some of the rules just changed on a daily basis after 9/11.

Kirk Caldwell I assume that you had to be in constant contact with the unions that represent your employees.

Peter Ingram They have been very cooperative throughout the time, but they are obviously representing the concerns of their members who are our employees, and so are we, and we don't always agree. One of the interesting initial debates was around face coverings. And I don't know if you remember at the beginning of all this, but the CDC's guidance was that healthy people shouldn't be wearing face coverings. The thinking was that it's likely to make you touch your face more because you're adjusting it and it can get moist, so you could make yourself sick. So we shouldn't wear face coverings was the guidance.

We have a lot of employees who were wanting to wear face coverings and, initially, based on the CDC guidelines, we were saying, "No, that's against our policy." Eventually, long before it became a recommendation to start wearing them, we relented and said, "Look, people aren't going to feel mentally comfortable just dealing with a bunch of strangers if we don't let them take what they view to be a protective measure even if the CDC hadn't yet gotten around to recommending it." Then of course it became CDC guidance later on. You and others implemented various orders around this.

The stay-at-home, work-from-home orders affected us a little bit less because we were designated as an essential industry. We have people—as do Hawaiian Electric and others—who have to be here to keep things moving. Mainly, it affected our administrative staff who had the ability to work remotely. To this day, if you look around our offices, it's sparsely populated even though we are now encouraged to return, what we're calling the phase we're in now. Not everyone has taken the encouragement at this point. But if you went over to our maintenance facility you would see the offices there are fuller; it's more front line–oriented. And of course, pilots can't work remotely; they have to be in the cockpit of the airplane. Flight attendants have to be in the airplane and airport agents have to be at the airport.

Kirk Caldwell The quarantine that the state implemented, if it had not been implemented, would we still see the same result at least short term? People not willing to fly?

Peter Ingram We still would have ended up dramatically reducing our schedule. Even if there were no quarantine restrictions or other travel restrictions, demand came dramatically down in other jurisdictions. Maybe not down 99 percent like we were down, but they came down 90 percent. So we would have had schedule reductions. I think what we would have seen is more of a ramp back up in the June/July period of 2020. Last summer, even around Memorial Day, people started traveling more, but for us that was delayed until October, when we got pretravel testing in place.

You talked about the meetings around opening up and that actually started with opening travel. I think we started having those meetings in May because the governor came out with the announcement that we would open up Neighbor Island travel starting June 15, 2020. At the time, my expectation was that we would closely follow with long-haul travel starting to open up, but that was when we saw the surge post–Memorial Day in California. Cases started rising again and I think that pushed everyone into a cautious mode. Unlike what you had in terms of the city restrictions being open and then closing again, we never got around to opening that long-haul flying, only Neighbor Island. We opened Neighbor Island June 15 to August 15, with no restrictions on travel including no testing restrictions. Then August 15, as the cases were rising on O‘ahu, we had the county mayors push aggressively for travel from O‘ahu to be restricted, which clamped things back down there again in terms of demand.

Kirk Caldwell What resources did you rely on with making decisions on how to position Hawaiian Airlines in the midst of a pandemic?

Peter Ingram We obviously were connected with the other carriers. One of the things, as competitive as we are in this business, we don't compete on safety. We collaborate on safety. The health of our guests and our teammates falls in the safety category. So there was plenty of sharing of information starting at the CEO level. There's been an ongoing industry conference call with our chief operating officer and our head of marketing with other senior leaders of the airlines. They're sharing best practices and what's going on, discussing policy, particularly federal policy.

We had a discussion on where we can get independent information on health and we ended up hiring a consulting physician to try and advise us on what was going on there and how we should think about things.

One of the things I realized pretty quickly was I couldn't be involved in every decision, so some of these things had to be delegated. I need to be plugged in, but you talk about eighteen hours a day. If you're trying to get too granular on some stuff, then you're going to miss entirely different things. Personally, my time at different phases was on one thing a lot and then a lot of checking in with my team who were focused on the other things. We went from having one senior officer meeting a week to having check-ins every day, just for half an hour, just so we all knew what each other was doing. But then we had to go and do things.

There was a period of time I ended up spending a fair amount of time with our finance and treasury team on some of the cash raising.

Communications was an important part of it. We like to make a lot of decisions in a collaborative consensus way. But when you're in a crisis like this, there comes a point where the most important thing is that there is a decision. And if you're the one with whom the buck stops in your organization, you've gotta just start making some of those calls and giving people clarity that this is the direction we're going—always with the caveat that forty-eight hours later we could get new information and be going in a different direction, but right now this is the direction we're going so people could get out and do it.

Business leaders from around the state converged in groups to start talking about how Hawai'i could survive and recover. One of the most active groups was through the Hawai'i Executive Collaborative (HEC), under the steersmanship of Duane Kurisu.

Kirk Caldwell When I see you, I think of a saying that I wish more city planners would follow, "To plan is human; to implement, divine." You literally knocked on our door and said, "Can we talk? We want to help you." When you showed up with the HEC, it was a sea change. How did this come about?

Duane Kurisu Thank you, Kirk. Hawai'i did not rise up to the crisis, but instead the crisis rose up to us. We in Hawai'i are a resilient people. When we join hands to protect our people and our turf, the best comes out of us. We stand second to nobody.

Those words are actually foundational for the Collaborative. The organization is living and working collaboratively with as many stakeholders as possible in creating the Hawai'i that we see in our heads and feel in our hearts. It's about rediscovering and protecting Hawai'i's soul in everything that we do. That is what makes us a special people. That is our strategic advantage over anyone and any place in the world. As such, we have a responsibility to share ourselves with the rest of the world. In this regard, I cannot think of a more appropriate person to honor than Nainoa Thompson, for his will and passion to commit his life to this responsibility and for his leadership with the Polynesian Voyaging Society in being the flashlight for the world.

So I think that it was instinctive that leaders in the HEC jumped into the fire when the crisis started incubating. It was putting things in action but it was in a significantly shorter time frame. For many of us, we were at war, and we worked and worried behind the scenes day and night.

There were some crossovers with others, including the governor's task force, to look at statewide solutions. There was a large and growing number of people involved with planning through the governor's office and it was getting more difficult to get our voice heard. So rightly or wrongly, we called on you to march to our own drum. I think that any plan that requires unified action by many people needs to show how we will win. Although we imagined it in the beginning, it is the part of our plan that never showed up until the pandemic matured and the tier system was adopted. We felt that with the pandemic we were in a state of crisis. And in a crisis, the public needs to be provided a picture of what the future would look like—when we can go back to living our lives in ways that we are accustomed to. We felt that we needed to find ways to take as much worry and fear out of people's lives now and in the future.

Of course, the issues surrounding the pandemic were unprecedented and who really would know what lay in front of us in the future, because we really can't predict the future. But in crisis, we need to bring comfort and relief from fear through our words and our commitment. A commitment to win. A commitment for hope that when we stand together and help each other go through these difficult times, we will be okay in the end.

Along the way, it was vital to get government involved. We could not do this in isolation because, at the end of the day, we need government for regulatory action, for implementing the law, and of course for signing relief checks. We recognized that we needed to work with someone who was similarly action-oriented and someone who would be willing to help break through the barriers of red tape. The first person that came to mind was you.

Early in the pandemic, the Hawai'i Executive Collaborative felt that our community's leaders in the COVID effort should be in front of people as much as possible. To that end, under the leadership of HEC executive director Lynelle Marble, we helped start and seed a weekday show online, in partnership with commentators Yunji de Nies and Ryan

Tsuji, together with *The Honolulu Star-Advertiser,* to help fill that need and to help bridge the communication void between State leadership and the general public. This show eventually became *Spotlight Hawaii* (podcast) for *The Honolulu Star-Advertiser.* And you were one of the first to be on the show. In times of crisis, every passing hour is an hour of turmoil and worry. With your help, I think this show contributed in bringing needed information and opinions, and in bringing clarity to the grave issues facing us during the early days of the pandemic.

Kirk Caldwell What does a win look like? If you know how you're going to win, you know how to get there too, right?

Duane Kurisu In visioning what normalcy in our lives would look like, a key tangible gauge was when restaurants and bars begin to open up. When things start opening up and people start shopping and visiting sit-down restaurants and bars, it would mean people felt safe, confident that most of the risks were mitigated and are comforted that the fears of the pandemic were largely behind us.

So it was not about restaurants opening. It was really about creating a pathway for building an environment of public confidence. Of course, the restaurants and retailers were already busy working on how they could open their doors for customers while keeping their employees safe. But there continued to be haziness and uncertainty from our policy makers on when and how things may start opening up. So during one of our weekly committee meetings with you early on, we decided to bring together leaders in the restaurant and retail industries.

Together with some of the Collaborative committee members, Chris Benjamin, CEO of Alexander & Baldwin, agreed to chair this ad hoc committee. We reached out to Tina Yamaki, president of the Retail Merchants of Hawaii; Sheryl Matsuoka, executive director of the Hawai'i Restaurant Association; and some other key leaders in the restaurant, bar, and retail industries and some owners of commercial real estate to come up with a collaborated plan. This group came up with a reopening strategy and the foundation for the tier system, which was first introduced by you during one of your midday public forums.

The core of it eventually became the tier system used by the state as its guide for reopening during the pandemic.

Your semiweekly public forums during the pandemic became the go-to place to introduce new ideas. While the Collaborative and The Omidyar Group provided support for aio Digital in their work with the DOH in building the contact tracing app, AlohaSafe Alert, there were few avenues available from the government side to let the public know that it was coming with the app to help alleviate the spread of COVID-19. Kirk, you welcomed AlohaSafe to make presentations several times. Because AlohaSafe was new and untested, you took some risk on having them on your show. But in the end, AlohaSafe became the most successful Apple and Google supported contract tracing app in the United States. AlohaSafe eventually became the default contact tracing app that all visitors were required to download during the pandemic. I think you should be acknowledged for your boldness in giving AlohaSafe a chance.

Then there is the story of Every1ne Hawaii, an action-oriented non-profit organization of emerging leaders, creatives, and influencers united in aloha to keep Hawai'i home. This organization placed a vital boots-on-the-ground approach to get people to use AlohaSafe. If you may recall, you allowed members of Every1ne Hawaii to be on your show to help Hawai'i residents understand the importance of AlohaSafe, and also to show them how to navigate the use of the app.

But all the while, there was something else that was brewing nationally and locally. Doctors from all over the United States were contacting my son, Robert Kurisu, a cofounder of Every1ne Hawaii, saying that unless everyone starts using face masks, they feared for themselves, for their fellow healthcare providers, that they were going to die. Some of his friends and friends of friends were doctors in New York and other major cities in hospitals in the middle of the worst times of the crisis. It was a chaotic, stressful, and scary time for all.

Every1ne Hawaii needed a forum. Every1ne Hawaii needed a base from which to start letting people know how important it was to use face masks and to teach them how to use face masks. So the first person they turned to for action was Kirk Caldwell. Sure enough, you provided them that forum and allowed them to be on your show. In fact, one of those guys on your show, Dr. Darragh O'Carroll, ended up being a regular on national television as a spokesperson for the face masks.

Kirk Caldwell Do you remember who came to be a spokesperson besides your son and Darragh O'Carroll? She got a gold medal at the Olympics. Your son brought Carissa Moore! She came, and she came with her sister and father, and she spoke. She was talking in the spirit of Duke Kahanamoku—she was channeling him—and it had a significant impact along with the other speakers.

Duane Kurisu Those presentations were moving, Kirk. And there were others like Zak Noyle and Kimo Kennedy, who played significant roles in helping to create that movement. I now remember that Sig Zane created a special face mask for you and that sparked others in the community to start making homemade face masks to help relieve the shortage of disposable masks at the time. I don't know if anyone realizes how significant this partnership was. At that very critical time, very few people nationally believed in face masks, except those in healthcare. The national movement for self-responsibility in using face masks started in Hawaiʻi right here at Honolulu Hale. It is awe-inspiring to witness what can be accomplished with pure will and commitment. I hope that one day history will be kind in recounting how many lives across the United States were saved because of Every1ne Hawaii and your willingness to partner with them when you were mayor in introducing face masks.

Kirk Caldwell CDC wasn't mandating the use of face masks, but even so the people of Hawaiʻi learned about the importance of using face masks to protect others from themselves. But the significant shortage of PPE and even if people were reaching out to different parts of the world to get the face masks, many were disappointed with unfulfilled orders due to a global shortage or the shipment of face masks that were substandard. This young group used their contacts and ingenuity to find a reputable source of face masks in China. I remember that they were supposed to have made an announcement during the press conference but then had trouble with the timing of getting the masks out from

China. They didn't come when they were supposed to and Hawaiian Airlines had to rearrange their schedule because the masks didn't show up on the tarmac at the right time. Once they came to the Hale to make the announcement, they were off and running on their own.

Duane Kurisu With the help of Peter Ingram, CEO of Hawaiian Airlines, and the Collaborative, they flew in two million masks from China. I can't remember what Peter and his staff did getting the charter flight to China and back with the face masks, but I know it was not easy. My opinion is that it was like carrying contraband out of China. The Chinese government, early in the pandemic, took control of all PPE being shipped outside of China.

They should have had a band playing when the Hawaiian Airlines flight landed on the tarmac as the airport fire trucks shot the plane with plumes of water in celebration. After all, this was two million face masks for Hawai'i that Hawai'i desperately needed but did not have.

Kirk Caldwell Then the group was out at Hale'iwa, West Side, Waialua, Wai'anae—in all these rural communities.

Duane Kurisu The Collaborative was not involved with the distribution. It was all done by the next generation guys with boots on the ground. It's funny. Somebody donated a cargo truck to them, and they painted it with the Every1ne Hawaii logo on it. You probably still see the truck on the road. It was this truck that transported face masks to rural areas on O'ahu where they distributed the masks for free. They partnered with other nonprofit groups for distribution to families for free, and you helped with some of those distribution efforts too. I remember seeing pictures of crates of the face mask being unloaded from a helicopter in Hilo, flown in by the Hawai'i National Guard, to take care of the emergency needs for the Big Island. Gives me chicken skin thinking about it now, with everyone, young and old, pitching in to help their friends and neighbors in time of need. Of course people were really thankful. You must be comforted reflecting on the fact that the public education on the importance of the use of face masks started at Honolulu Hale.

Kirk Caldwell Dr. Fauci would say, next to the vaccine, the best thing to do is wear a face mask. No doubt. I forgot all about the face masks in the early days of all these initiatives. The City and County of Honolulu was also rushing to get face masks—we were believers and we purchased them through sources in China. We wanted N95s and we had our fire department guys test them, and they weren't N95s. First Hawaiian Bank was able to solve the problem.

Duane Kurisu Whether it was political or whether it was to fulfill shortages among its own people, China wasn't allowing any of the face masks to get out. So my son, Robert, worked with a friend who does a lot of business in China. My understanding is that his friend helped repackage the face masks to meet the prevailing Chinese laws, which allowed them to be loaded onto the waiting Hawaiian Airlines jet for shipment to Hawai'i. I think this is what caused the delay on the shipment that you and I talked about earlier.

Kirk Caldwell There was also this major HEC effort centered around food distribution in our more rural communities that made a significant difference for families struggling to make ends meet.

Duane Kurisu In that case, it was really Micah Kane, CEO of Hawai'i Community Foundation (HCF), and Randy Hiraki, owner of Commercial Plumbing. It was Micah and you who had the first conversation. Then Randy stepped in because he believed that even in the most difficult times, you didn't shut down the construction workers. Randy felt that the construction companies and their workers continued to make money while many people in other industries were shut down with no work. So he said, "Let's call on people in the construction industry to share in what we have." He came to talk story with me and I said, "Okay, let's go."

We are blessed to live in a place like Hawai'i, where the people are the most generous and empathetic people in the world. In watching and listening to the people who were volunteering and giving out the food, I think they probably gained more out of giving the food than the people getting the food. You were out there too, Kirk, and you saw and heard the plight of those who needed help, and the satisfaction and generosity of those who provided help.

Kirk Caldwell I saw a couple driving a nice brand-new Lexus but needing food because they were unemployed for the first time in their lives and had no money and had never asked for a handout. They talked about the shame they felt. But they gathered up their courage and came. You gave them hope.

Duane Kurisu I give them probably the most credit for coming down. Brand-new Lexus; you could surmise that both husband and wife were laid off from executive jobs in the hospitality, restaurant, or retail industry. Instinctively, you say to yourself, hey, you gotta do what you gotta do to feed your family.

Micah Kane Ron Mizutani, Hawai'i Foodbank, came into the mix in coordination through our food security program. He was a big driver. We did the first one out in Waipi'o, and it was tough. You went out there. The lineup of cars—people were waiting four, five, six hours. And then to be able to bring it into the stadium, finding a way to do it more efficiently to a point where their wait was maybe an hour.

Kirk Caldwell We learned a lot. Did some of that come out of the ALICE (Asset Limited, Income Constrained, Employed) Report?

Micah Kane We were very fortunate that this community understood the ALICE state of the union of Hawai'i. Going into the pandemic knowing that just about one out of every two families is one paycheck away from a financially catastrophic situation. It's pretty common sense that when you're hit by a pandemic like that what the magnitude of the hit might be. Your concern goes through the roof pretty quickly. And you saw it. The faces that you see when you're there are not people that want to take a handout. They're not used to doing that. In fact, they're very uncomfortable about doing that. They're used to helping other people, not asking for help themselves.

Kirk Caldwell It wasn't people coming in busted up cars. They're driving nice cars, but they didn't have a job and very limited income. They had rent and mortgages to pay and families to feed.

Micah Kane And very capable people. It's a real hit on their morale. Hard for them.

Kirk Caldwell Were there times when you wanted to give up? This is too hard. Too much bureaucracy. Too much ego.

Micah Kane No, there was never a time in any of our dealings with any one of the county leaders that I felt there wasn't a willing partner throughout the pandemic. What I hoped would have happened is that there would have been a common framework by which we all were looking through as we rolled out our various initiatives. It evolved kind of at the end, but it took way too long to get to.

Kirk Caldwell The things I wish were different… I wish we had different leadership at the DOH at the beginning of the pandemic. In the early days that was a real struggle for our administration. And then on top of that trying to get the governor to act instead of listening to [Bruce] Anderson or [Sarah] Park. In some ways it's admirable that he listens to his cabinet leaders, he trusts them, but I think it kept us from acting quicker and resulting in better outcomes. And for me, I think I should have pushed harder.

Micah Kane I think you pushed pretty hard, Mayor. It's hard for me to be critical not knowing what people are dealing with. You just trust that people are making the right decisions based on the information they have. From our lens though, it looked like we could have saved a lot of small businesses had we acted faster. That is something that is part of our culture that I'm not sure we're going to see come back too quickly.

I think it's dangerous to Monday morning quarterback yourself or others right now. I feel like the best opportunity we have is looking forward. Taking the muscle that we developed and not letting it get atrophied again. A lot of people are burned out by the different groups that have surfaced to try to continue to solve some of the issues that we're facing. I think we have to stick with it. I think we have to bring all of those forces together because there's different factions in our community that need to coalesce so that people are more efficient in the use of their time and their resources. It's on the table for us right now, but I see it starting to atrophy as our economy comes back and as we address the challenges facing our tourism industry.

Ron Mizutani (Hawai'i Foodbank) So it was a Friday afternoon, Mayor. I had this vision. You know that we need to get food out to a much larger population. People who don't even know how to raise their hands. And I'd seen some video of these food distributions happening on the US Mainland, but we never did it here. Not at that intense level. So I knew it would take money, I knew it would take a lot of collaboration not with just the private sector but also with government. I called Micah Kane and we got on the phone with you folks and I said, "Give me a weekend to put something together. I'll come back with you guys and we'll figure this out. I just need two days." Pam Witty-Oakland (director of the City Department of Community Services) said, "Let's do it." Micah said, "Whatever you need. We'll get the money. Just give us your strategy on how you want to do this. Location, etc. And we'll get it done." That's how it happened. Over a weekend. I sat down and put all my thoughts on paper, what I visualized we could execute with a tremendous army, but again, all that required funding, which I did not have.

My budget at the time was $400,000 to purchase food but donations came to a halt. From our stores, from our partners, from our community—everybody was just taking care of their own. So what was a $400,000 budget for annual food purchase, I knew we would not be able to do it. And that's when I came to you and Micah. Peter Ho and the HCF and Bank of Hawai'i responded with that two-million-dollar gift.

I think I've shared with you and the public before, every dime of that two million dollars—one million dollars from the City, and one million dollars from HCF and the Bank of Hawai'i—every single dime of it went to the purchasing of food. Not a single penny went to the food bank's administrative costs, operational costs—nothing. Every single dime of it went to food to go back to the community. That was a commitment that I made to you, to Pam, and to Micah. We would find a way to pay our bills later. Let's get food in the hands of those who need it.

That was in April. Our first distribution was a week and a half later. It was an absolute nightmare. Waipi'o Soccer Complex. We were so new to it. We gathered food partners and volunteers and we just came up with this plan. We learned along the way. We got way better at it.

But the reality is, this was done with an army of volunteers, not just from our private sector partners, but also, later on, Duane Kurisu and the gang from the construction industry stepped up in a huge way. It really came down to people still willing to be a part of the community even though they were losing their jobs. We had people who were losing their jobs volunteering, distributing food, and then jumping in their car and then getting in line. That's the specialness of our islands; the humanitarian effort that we all saw come together in a very short time.

Besides philanthropy and the foundations, the administration was huge in these executions of food distributions, which eventually made their way to rural areas and then pop-ups. We really worked closely with the administration, and, of course, our private sector partners, to get it done, but this didn't happen by chance. This took a lot of effort and *kōkua* and just believing in each other. It was awesome to be a part of.

Kirk Caldwell Could you describe that first food distribution?

Ron Mizutani I'm getting emotional thinking about it. I never lost that feeling. We never realized the impact we would have. Nor did we realize the scope of what our community was experiencing. There's no dignity waiting in line for six, seven hours for food. There's a tremendous amount of humility to that, so I would remind our incredible volunteers, many who came back for every single distribution, that there's courage going on today. People are raising their hand for the first time in their lives. They may not make eye contact with you, they may not say a word, you may see tears, people may not even say thank you. Raising your hand because you're hungry, there's a stigma to it. I'm not comparing it to domestic violence, but it's very similar where the shame factor is very real.

And when you see cars lined up the way they did, and some of them absolutely in tears leaving, thanking you, because both spouses or entire families in some cases were without jobs. Pulling up in a brand-new BMW and you go, *Wow, this is real.* It's easy to see a Tesla and say, *Really? You need this?* And the reality is yeah, they did.

Kirk Caldwell It was incredible that you were able to pull this food distribution program together in just a week and a half.

Ron Mizutani Some of it was existing relationships. Some of it was brand-new relationships, including the Hawai'i Farm Bureau. Brian Miyamoto—I knew of his work, but I'd never met him. I cold called him that weekend, by the way. I was drafting this plan and I said, "Brian, I'm Ron from Hawai'i Foodbank. I know the farmers are hurting right now. Our restaurants are going to be closing if they haven't already, and the hotels are certainly following close by. How do I get the farmers to keep on farming?" And that became an incredible friendship.

It's all about relationships in Hawai'i and before you know it we had a core group of food providers who became dear friends, and we were in this fight together. That just created new friends, new relationships, and it was a ripple effect because people were seeing the good work that we were doing. They weren't there to make a dime. Truly, the farmers appreciated what we did. I had this vision. We need produce and we don't have any. So how do we get produce? We get it from our farmers. I told Miyamoto from the get-go, "I'll commit $200,000 of this two-million-dollar gift—dollars that we have from the city and HCF—$200,000 from Hawai'i Foodbank money to buy just produce and let's see where this goes." And by the time I left, we had purchased over $1.5 million of locally grown produce. That in itself is a great story to be told because it kept the farmers going and it was through our efforts—the

City and HCF—that this happened.

At the end, not only did we serve our community fresh produce—and I include beef in that because that's produce, anything that was locally produced by our farmers. Fish, that's a whole different story, right? We just got more creative and as the days went by, the months went by, we found different ways to get food to people offering quality and healthy options for families that needed it.

Kirk Caldwell Ron, you kept those farmers farming. You put money back into their pockets. Otherwise they would be hurting just like everyone else. You provided them more security.

Ron Mizutani A few of the farmers called personally and said, "Thank you for keeping our business alive. And thank you for keeping our employees working." It was a small investment, but it was a large investment because it started the conversation. It reminded all of us if we want to be resilient as a community our farmers need to be a part of that conversation and at the table. I hope that once this pandemic is pau that continues to be a focus. We need to invest in them because when we needed them most, they were there.

Kirk Caldwell It's important what you're saying, Ron. Can we talk a little bit about the fish distribution program too? As you know, our fishing fleet and our local fishermen lost a big part of their market when the tourism industry shut down. What the food bank did helped them continue to cover their expenses and keep an industry alive that we all depend on.

Ron Mizutani It was the same model that we used for the farmers. Now granted, fish is a whole different product when it comes to keeping them refrigerated and all the safety aspects that come with that. A little more tricky. I told our team, "Please don't tell me why we can't do it. Tell me how we can do this." And before you know it, we had fresh fish in people's hands on a weekly basis. Fish that would have not been caught—literally, boats, like farmers, were tied up. And we knew this was not going to be forever once the restaurants return to business and hotels open, but they needed that little boost. We certainly didn't put in anywhere near the money that we put into the farmers, but we started that conversation and we too committed out of the gate $50,000 to our fishing industry. And I think after that people understood that this is an important industry to keep going. In fact, it's a multibillion dollar industry that went silent once those restaurants and hotels closed.

Kirk Caldwell Incredible story. From the point of fish being caught to being distributed to keeping it fresh—there's a lot of moving parts and yet you got them all in place and working really well.

Ron Mizutani It took a lot of creativity and a lot of collaboration—and I hate to use that word too much because it's overused. But it really did take a team effort, problem-solving, and—lord knows we did have some missteps along the way—but nobody ever got sick and, in fact, it became where people became spoiled. They were getting *kalua* pig and fresh *poke*, and in distribution lines people would say, "Eh, what happened this week? We nevah had kalua pig?"

Those are the kind of relationships that make a difference. I called Halms and said, "Look, let's give you business. How much kalua pig can you give me for X amount of dollars?" Again, they weren't trying to make money. They were just trying to keep their business going and all of them appreciated what we did as a food bank and we just duplicated and mirrored that across the entire state where all the other food banks were doing similar things. We just did it on a larger level here on O'ahu because of our population.

Kirk Caldwell I think your model and what you did kept the infrastructure of farming and fishing in place at a time where we would have lost a portion of it and when we return to a healthy economy it wouldn't be there. You gave them that lifeline to continue to operate so they would be there later. That's an unwritten story. But those who know, those who you threw lines out to, they understand that they are around today because you provided an opportunity that wouldn't have been there. They'd have to sell their boats and get rid of farm equipment, but they're able to pay their loans and balance their books because of you.

Ron Mizutani It wasn't just me. It was a lot of people. I went back to some of the out-of-the-box thinking that came from watching my grandparents, my father, my mom, my cousins, and my sister—everybody else trying to figure it out after Iniki. Living in tents, no water, no ice, no phone service—I lived it with them and watched it. I was on O'ahu at the time, but I visited frequently to see them, make sure that people weren't going cuckoo. Whew, if Iniki had happened on O'ahu, we'd see crisis and chaos. But we lived through our share of crisis with COVID.

Kirk Caldwell You mentioned the construction industry and Duane Kurisu and Randy Hiraki's effort to continue your food distribution program into more rural areas. Could you talk about that a little bit? And how that came together at the end of summer, the early fall, and right before Thanksgiving of 2020. I know that one of their distributions was taking place on the North Shore right before a hurricane started to impact O'ahu, and it still went ahead because they wanted to distribute food to as many people as possible.

Ron Mizutani I think that just talking to Randy, Duane, and those in the industry, the Kobayashi Group, and everybody else that continued to work, they were considered essential and they understood that their men and women on the line were continuing to bring home a paycheck. It was their way of saying, "You know what? We need to do our part as well."

When Randy and Duane called, I gave them a quick tour of the food bank and they asked, "How can we help?" I said, "Well, we got another food distribution planned and it takes a tremendous amount of funding and volunteers," and they didn't even hesitate. "Let's do it. How much do you need?" And I wanted to mirror what we had been doing with the City and HCF. Our funding was running out with that, but clearly the virus wasn't going anywhere and there still were needs, so they stepped in right at a time when we needed a little more funding.

And they were huge. It was a huge part of our mission of survival for another month and change. They stepped in right at an opportune time. And I think, and I know, they got a lot out of it. They came with their volunteers in their construction uniforms—and talk about people who are efficient. They were setting up—setup sometimes took us an hour—they did it in thirty-five minutes because they know how to work hard. At the end, you could see in their faces, they realized the impact that they were having not only distributing food, but seeing the faces, talking to the folks—some of them their own friends. It was a huge lift for their own teams to be grateful but also to be grateful for the city and state that we live in and that there are people who are willing to help when we need it most. Their help came at a time when the food bank really needed it.

Kirk Caldwell I saw that. These are big men, tough guys, and they worked very efficiently and quickly.

Ron Mizutani Very emotional too. There were guys who came up to me after they were done—and they were hulking, muscular, young men—and said, "Thank you for having us here. That was amazing." Again, it was all about relationships, partnerships, and friendships that we had established with the City and some of our food partners. We expanded to include even more food partners and provided a different menu to those who were in line. In the venues, some of them were private, some of them were schools—Windward Community College, Leeward Community College—and then our pop-up distributions. We thought, *We gotta do this even better. How can we touch people out on the North Shore, Lāʻie?* And we got even more creative by having these smaller pop-up distributions that became a part of what we did.

All the distributions were impactful for those who could make it to Hālawa, but not everybody had a ride to Hālawa, let alone have the mobility to head out to Hālawa, and that's why we went to them—out in Lāʻie and Kāneohe. We just did some amazing work and, again, thank you for always finding a way to get it done. I can't tell you how many times your park permit people just said, "What do you need?" I said, "I need a park." "Okay, what time?" And all the permit processes were honored, but it was expedited because the needs were so great.

Kirk Caldwell It's amazing. You went big and small. And you were very creative in terms of trying to get food to where it needed to be and in the most convenient way to distribute it. It was amazing to see you turn on a dime and be really creative with your solutions.

Ron Mizutani It wasn't just creativity though, Mayor. Keep in mind, we never increased our staff ever, during the pandemic. In fact, we lost a few people. In the end, what drove us and drove our team the most was continuing to focus on respect. Respect those in line. And if we stay true to our mission, we'll be fine. I'm not going to say that we didn't have any breakdowns in our own place, but as far as execution, it took creativity, it took funding, but it also took us understanding what role we were playing at that time.

Health vs. Education

The closure of schools and the transition to online learning was a major impact on both public and private school systems. Like businesses, the issues were complex. It was more than facing compromised teaching and learning. It was also about the deterioration of family units; the lack of resources, devices, and access to the internet; and for some children, a concern for their safety, the lack of adult supervision, and even making sure they were getting enough food. Teachers also faced the challenges of teaching remotely. The stories from 'Iolani School and the DOE were dramatically different in terms of how these organizations fared and what they were up against.

Tim Cottrell ('Iolani School) It's a huge detriment not to have kids go to school in person. We were early in our preparation to be online and we were also one of the first schools to say that being online is not good for kids and that it is imperative to get back to in-person learning as soon as safely possible. That was August 2020. We wanted to return to campus for our normal start of school. We had just completed summer school online, so we were ready to open on campus, and then the case count in the state grew exponentially. We had to pause for some weeks but we did open in September for all grades and got everybody back to in-person learning. This was absolutely from the perspective that it is developmentally damaging to take children out of the social context in which they learn. A lot of their social-emotional development goes on in the "herd" of young people who are growing up together. And this varies for different ages. Young children are different from adolescents, who are different from young adults, but, every one of those groups needs peers around them. I think it gets more and more important as kids get older. If you ask a teenager what their most important thing in the world is most of them will say, "My friends." It is that important. The lockdown experience was isolating and very hard on kids.

Academically, however, online is fairly good. You can teach algebra online. That's not a huge hurdle. But that's not everything the experience of school is about. We could ensure students would continue to receive good instruction in their classes and stay on schedule academically. However, the shutdown came with a huge cost socially, in terms of isolation.

Then, students didn't come back to an ideal situation. They had to wear masks and face shields, wash their hands every time they entered and exited a classroom, sit outside a lot, eat outside—there were a lot of restrictions. However, at the end of the day, as I think educators would have predicted, the students were willing to do pretty much anything that would allow them to be back on campus, learning and interacting with their friends.

Returning to campus in September 2020 with these new PPE protocols presented new challenges for our faculty as well. Initially, it was hard to teach with a mask and shield, so we provided our faculty with wireless microphones to amplify their voices. We also instituted additional days off throughout the school year to avoid burnout. We added many more four-day weeks and found that our community was just as productive, if not more, by adding in these additional days to reenergize and regroup.

Kirk Caldwell From the littlest ones?

Tim Cottrell Yes, we created little, teeny face shields all the way up to adult sizes for the different age groups.

Kirk Caldwell That is resilience.

Tim Cottrell There was so much undermining of science during that time and so much inconsistency. It's still kind of continuing now. People fixate on the one case of something and that's like the biggest news. But statistically, maybe it's not. It's just news, our world of clickbait. Some people were social distancing, some people were something else, some people were focusing on another thing, and if you try to do all of those things you really couldn't run a school. It is impossible to have a school where kids are six feet apart all the time. Nobody has the square footage to do that. So if we can't do that, then create an environment in which the main source of transmission, through the breath, is highly mitigated. This was the basis on which we prioritized different prevention strategies and created a plan that allowed us to safely be on campus.

We were fortunate to have a lot of experts who we could talk to and who were willing to review our safety plan. We said, "Okay, we're going to do PPE in an incredibly rigorous, diligent, and extreme way, and we're going to make sure our kids wash their hands a lot, all day long." With that, we were pretty much there in terms of safety without social distancing inhibiting the ability to operate as a school. And we added in a lot more. We generated QR codes for students to scan and placed them at every seat. We could track and trace everybody who sat anywhere, anytime during the day. We put air purifiers in our rooms. We bought the UV room cleaners that hospitals use. We worked to address everything we could.

In retrospect, this could pretty much have been accomplished using a face mask and a face shield, which is less than a ten-dollar investment per student, and washing your hands a lot. Ultimately, that's all it took to have students on campus in a safe way as long as they bought into the restrictions. Our students were disciplined with the PPE protocols the whole year, and although COVID existed in the larger community and our students interacted in this space, we had no cases of on-campus transmission of COVID during the entire 2020–21 school year.

The other thing that made a huge difference was our decision to maximize the use of outdoor spaces throughout campus. We put up twenty large tents all over our campus, which allowed everyone to eat outdoors and provided a space where our students could spend their free periods. The tents are now so popular we have pressure to find a way to keep some of them permanently.

If there's a shame in it all, it's that there was an accessible and cost-effective solution for everybody to stay in school. You didn't have to be ʻIolani and buy air purifiers for every single room or some other prevention measure that was cost-prohibitive. Those measures did help people feel a high degree of safety around them, so in the emotional domain all those things were important to get everybody back to work. But, in practical terms regarding safety, we just had to make sure all of our students and faculty were good about wearing their face masks and face shields and washing their hands a lot.

The comparison between what ʻIolani was able to do and what the public DOE was able to do was stark.

Christina Kishimoto (Hawaiʻi DOE) Think about how large we are. If you're in a gymnasium breaking down millions of individual pieces of PPE to send out to three hundred schools and trying to figure out how to transport all those items—you usually have a professional team that does that. Well, it's my team doing that. It's my team trying to figure it out and going around to check sites, such as the feeding sites. My job at that point was to be a cheerleader while also rolling up my sleeves. I knew they would do a great job, and I thank them.

Doing that from afar, you can't give anyone hugs and everyone's covered up. Just thanking them and waving to parents and saying, "It's going to be okay," "How are your kids?" and "How are you doing?" So, there was all of that. Aloha was something we had to give too because as educators we lead from the heart, but at the same time we're trying to figure out how to feed our children and distribute PPE. We immediately went into counting devices. Literally, going into school buildings, breaking down laptop cards. How many devices have a camera for instruction? So it's not just the device that's portable, but it has to have a camera.

We set up distribution sites all over the state for families to pick up a device. Now not only do you have to get them registered to that family, but you also now have to have safety features on a device to give to a child. We weren't set up that way and all of a sudden we're trying to figure out how to procure the safety features that we need to make sure we adhere again to federal and state law for devices that go home. All of this is quite complicated, and we realized we had a shortage of devices. Ideally, we needed ninety thousand new devices for our high-poverty kids. We had over a hundred thousand but the quality of these devices was a problem. We had old devices in a number of schools and so if we were going to truly give everyone a quality device, we needed about ninety thousand. I had stated we would need to purchase about thirty-five thousand to forty thousand devices, but that was the minimum. If I didn't have those devices, I would have kids who weren't learning at home because they would have no way to connect.

Georgette Deemer Were those devices iPads or phones?

Christina Kishimoto A combination of things. Mostly laptops and iPads. Primarily, Chromebooks. Those were the three types of devices. A phone was not sufficient.

Kirk Caldwell Who's going to train people on how to use these devices?

Christina Kishimoto Not just teachers, but the parents and grandparents need support—the aunties that were home with the kids suddenly. So, I brought my team together and said, "We need a help desk for families. I need multiple languages on that help desk." And my team said to me, "We're overwhelmed with the current help desk for our employees who haven't worked remotely, haven't worked in this way."

So I called Su Shin from Hawaiian Telcom and said, "You have a help desk system that you run. I need you to partner with me. Can you handle one for parents? Oh, and by the way, I have a minimum of six to seven language groups that are required, including really hard, difficult-to-find language groups like our Micronesian languages. While it's a small number of parents, they're the ones that needed the most help." And she says to me, "We will figure this out, Christina," and in a week's time we had the design for the help desk and a few weeks later she had everyone hired. We had my help desk here working with their help desk and we had a parent help desk."

Kirk Caldwell I don't think anyone knows about this extraordinary effort and partnership.

Christina Kishimoto I'm at the legislature, saying, "Folks—food, help desk, PPE. I need help!" And now we're going into an economic situation. "Well, what do you need?" I think I asked for $135 million of emergency support, but I told them what that was for and all of it was justified, and they had me come back five different times, five hearings.

So not only am I running around from food distribution places to distributing PPEs to figuring out these corporate partnerships, I'm now mandated to go to five hearings. I'm in the Hawaii State Capitol building that's shut down also, so I must be escorted in. After five hearings and the legislature closes, I get the phone call. "We've made a decision." Zero dollars. Zero dollars!

I have laptops on hold from the Mainland, and you know what the company says to me? "I can't hold this for you anymore. I have a waitlist of districts and I can deliver this down the street. Sorry, you lost them." We lost our entire order. We were checking laptops that were five, six, seven, eight years old to see if they would work.

They gave me zero dollars and I made a call maybe an hour after I got that news and said, "Are you kidding me? You gave zero dollars to our children. You know what's going to happen? I'm going to name you and the fact that you gave zero dollars." And everyone I was in the room with—and I don't know if you remember this, Kirk—within hours of closing the legislature they called an emergency hearing. Within twenty-four hours, they give me $6 million of the $135 million or so that I needed.

And I told them, "Keep it. Do not throw pennies at my children. I'm sorry, I don't want it." It's not that $6 million is pennies, right? People might listen to that and say it's $6 million, but it wasn't enough. I needed a minimum of $36 million just to hold the line with the ones that were broken. The governor, to his credit, turned around and said, "Spend the $36 million and I will find it for you."

We spent the money internally and a few weeks later, to his credit, he took state CARES money. He took it back from the legislature, he issued me exactly the minimum I needed—that $36 million—and he transferred it over to us, and we paid that bill. Now that's still with a $24 million food service bill that I was in the red on—you know, it was insane. It felt like we were just hanging on. I can't produce money, I can't generate taxes, I can't make any of those decisions. What I can do is help when a child is saying, "I need food, I need PPE, and I need a device because I don't own a computer. Oh, and by the way, we don't have internet/cable because we can't afford it."

We purchased seventeen thousand hot spots overnight by working with partners and saying, "Give me as many as you have," and we paid internet/cable bills for families to do this. We kept telling the State, "Look, we're the DOE. We don't solve connectivity, we don't pay internet/cable bills, but we must do this. Tell me what you want me to do." And then what's the next news we get? Legislature took $100 million out of our budget in the middle of all this.

Kirk Caldwell So instead of giving you additional money, they took money away?

Christina Kishimoto They took money away to balance the state budget or whatever they put it towards. And I had the promise from Senator Dela Cruz and others that that was going to be a temporary budget cut—and here we are, this session is closed and they made it a permanent budget cut. So $100 million lost last year, $100 million lost this year (2021); it's all cumulative. It feels a little biblical. "Go make brick with straws" is exactly how I would describe this year.

And it shouldn't be that hard. This is our community. You're not doing this for me, you're doing it for our children.

Kirk Caldwell So you got the hot spots and you're paying for students' internet/cable—that's amazing.

Christina Kishimoto We made an agreement with the cable company to buy the packages, so the hot spot came with the package. So we're not taking a bill from a family—we're giving them a hot spot that has a prepaid package. We had families with tears in their eyes thanking us: "You give us a device, you give us the hot spot, and that meant the world to us."

Kirk Caldwell Now you've got the teachers who must teach under a new mode. You have thirteen thousand teachers and they're no longer sitting in a classroom.

Christina Kishimoto Some of them were trying to teach on the phone because they were intimidated to teach online. So now we're pairing teachers up with other teachers who are comfortable, and the teachers, to their credit, on their own, created PD (professional development) hubs—I mean, it was impressive. Teachers who knew how to do distance teaching could teach others. They created their own teams while the DOE system itself created some PD programs and that's how we made it happen. It was really all the teachers; an all hands on deck, let's figure this out. And then we started, of course, the 2020 school year nine days late to do nine days of PD training on distance learning, which is the most PD they've ever gotten. But think about the miracle of a system that doesn't do distance teaching except in some select small spots through E-school and things like that, having every last teacher receive nine days of PD training on distance learning, distance teaching. That wouldn't have happened if it wasn't for the pandemic. So when you think about some of the good things that happened, if we had to negotiate that, it probably would never have happened. It would have been teacher opt-in. Now everyone was saying, "We gotta do this. We're on board," and so we agreed to that. And that was an easy lift with the unions to say, "Look, we need this." We were all in agreement—we needed to do this.

Kirk Caldwell So, the teachers through professional development start to learn how to teach online while at the same time you have the reality of younger kids trying to learn online. It's different than in a classroom and trying to adjust for that... You probably had kids that just didn't show up.

Christina Kishimoto We had attendance issues, 22 percent chronic absenteeism for this past year, so that's a 6–7 percent increase in chronic absenteeism. That's quite significant. It's a lot of instructional time lost. That doesn't count the kids who were online who weren't really paying attention.

And kids were trying to figure out what to do, calling their teacher: "I can't get on. What do I do?" And the teacher's trying to figure it out: "I don't know what to tell you." We had the help desk working, we had a huge spike all year long of help desk assistance that had to be on-demand for instruction to continue to happen. And you can't have a child on a screen for six hours. As adults, we can't be on a screen for six hours, so think about the quality of instruction. We're going to spend forty minutes here, we're going to do group work, we're going to shut this down, you're going to do these assignments, and you're going to check back in—you know, it's all spotty instruction and everybody did their best, but it was very, very difficult for everyone. Lots of instructional time was lost.

You have teachers saying, "Don't forget before you start school, even though you're online, you still got to brush your teeth and get out of your pajamas." They're on the screen. "And hey, don't forget, comb your hair." We had all of those kinds of things and for the first time not only were kids learning from home—when you think about kids in poverty, they now were exposing other people to what home was like. So kids were doing things like trying to cover the screen a little bit with a piece of paper, just showing their face. Some of them were holding babies and feeding the baby while they're on. We saw everything of that community. You have a parent in the back yelling, "When are you going to be done with class? I've got to get to the supermarket." That's not to disparage or discredit parents who did try to figure this out. The private space now became public. You know, the reality of home. *

CHAPTER 4

The Dreaded Second Surge

Kirk Caldwell We opened everything up by the end of May and then we started seeing cases going back up. First, it was ten or twenty. Then it was thirty. We locked down, the first time, under thirty-three, and now there's over thirty. There's fifty, eighty. So that's May, June, July. Then we're having 150.

Because Oʻahu doesn't have a health department, we formed a medical advisory panel. They were advising us, saying, "You opened up too quickly. You didn't listen to us and now you see these cases. You gotta start doing things to go the other way."

Libby Char (Hawaiʻi DOH) By then we had the medical group meeting regularly and we were having discussions in the afternoon about what should we open up, what was reasonable, how did it work. Even amongst the medical group, some were more conservative than others with the thought that we should wait two weeks in between actions. And it sounds very easy and reasonable to do on paper, but again, there has to be that realization that this is the medical public health perspective—there are other factors that have to be weighed into the overall decision.

And I think there was some frustration that we felt things were opening up too quickly, rather than opening something and sitting for two weeks. That's the incubation period. See how it goes and then make another move, then another move.

You were getting a lot of pressure from the business side especially, and even some of the larger business healthcare side too, to move a little bit faster. So understandably you were kind of in a difficult position.

Whatever you did, someone's unhappy. Yeah, the feeling was that you were moving too quickly and then once one thing opened and another thing opened, the businesses were jumping all over it: *Hey, you let this guy open. What about us?* And it was just like dominoes, everything was open again. Like in a few weeks, everything popped open again.

Kirk Caldwell So we opened up and then we started seeing a greater number of cases. I don't know if you have any theories. The thing that troubled me the most was just the visuals of people at the beaches. Fourth of July, every Saturday and Sunday. And not just local beaches, but even Waikīkī Beach became like a local beach—huge numbers of people under pop-up tents and others, no masks, no physical distancing, no nothing. I don't know if cases came from that, but one theory I have is that that attitude on the beach created this attitude that they carried with them everywhere, so even at home they gathered. They didn't always go to the beach, but big gatherings in their backyards. Where did this spread come from as we opened up?

Libby Char At the time things were happening, we didn't have as much knowledge about the virus as we do now. So we're making what we thought was the best decision based on the knowledge we had at the time. And outdoors should have been safe. I think some of the unintended consequence of that though was opening one venue conveyed an attitude or an unspoken message that we're opening up again, so we must be over this. It must be safe now. And like you said, if we can do this at the beach, why can't we do this in the backyard? And I think there were a lot of social gatherings and that attitude was kind of pervasive, so they were having large social gatherings, lots of people crowded together, not wearing masks. And I think that's where we started really seeing cases go up.

And after that Fourth of July weekend there were a lot of people congregating. Outdoor activities and beaches should have been safe, but people were gathering pretty tightly packed even though it was outdoors. That conveyed a higher risk. But it was really that unspoken messaging that went out that I think was the wrong message. Not intended.

But when we opened up a certain thing like hiking, beaches, parks, people kind of felt like, *Okay, we're done!* And that attitude carried forth into parties, gatherings, graduations.

Kirk Caldwell In August, Statehood Day, which must have been around the third week in August, Dr. Jon Dworkin told me he set up a time for me to go to the hospital to meet doctors, nurses, and others to see what's happening in the hospital. On that day, we had 355 cases. And I went to the hospital—you can tell when people are frightened and stressed—the doctors, the nurses, the orderlies, the people cleaning, everyone just had big eyes and looked very, very worried.

I saw people with COVID lying under clear shower curtains. I thought, *What is that? Did they die?*

No, you put it over them so when they're breathing it doesn't spread through the air with COVID. Every bed was like that. They must have gone to some bath store. And then I went up to the COVID ward and saw all the beds full and they were converting an additional floor to another COVID ward and they told me, "You know, Mayor, if you don't do something pretty soon it's going to be LA and New York. They're going to be in the hallways." And then they put a triage tent in front of Queen's and they actually put a tent outside Emergency where the ambulances came in. And they said, "You gotta shut down."

Libby Char I think I picked you up that day and drove you to the hospital. We thought it would be good for you to have an opportunity to see what it was like for the healthcare folks and get a different perspective. We went to the hospital and we met with Dr. Honda. We didn't even go into the ICU. We went into the ER, we went to the COVID unit, and we didn't go into any of the rooms, but we stood in the hall and we talked to the doctors and nurses and the respiratory therapists and the people that were taking care of frontline COVID patients. And I think it was palpable to know that on the other side of that door, or that wall, was somebody who was lying in a bed because they were sick enough with COVID that they needed to be in the hospital.

Down in the ER, there was someone who had been intubated and was on a ventilator. In order to limit the spread of COVID, they would pull a plastic sheet over the patient. I think it was very visually striking to you because I remember seeing your reaction, and I remember you commenting about it several times after. To see somebody lying in bed, on a ventilator, with a piece of plastic sheeting pulled up all the way head to toe over them. You'd think that would be a shroud of a dead person.

Kirk Caldwell That's what it was, the feel of death. Like death was here in this room.

Libby Char And to think that you're standing twenty feet away, looking through a door at that person—you could reach out and touch them. And I know that had a big effect on you because you kept mentioning it.

Kirk Caldwell Did it have an effect on you—you, as a doctor—when you see that?

Libby Char It was a critically ill patient, so that wasn't something unknown to me but I know that was really significant for you. We went upstairs to talk to the doctors and nurses as they came out of the patient rooms, and they were telling you what they were seeing and what their day was like. Some of them remarked they had a woman in this room and her husband was in that room, and no family members could visit. You saw the fatigue that they were feeling, dealing with this day after day after day with the unspoken question, *When is this going to stop?* They were all working overtime and they were just exhausted and there was no end in sight.

Kirk Caldwell I told Jonathan that seeing that person under the shower curtain was dramatic for me but the other thing is looking at the faces of those who I talked to, starting with Dr. Honda, and all those people. They had that look. You know you can tell when someone is concerned. A little frightened, tired but frightened. You can sense when someone is like, this is serious, this is not the standard thing. And they had that look, that feeling, all of them. And I felt we were on the verge of a crisis, we were on the verge of an Italy or New York City where people are going to be in the hallways—and it was going to happen in the next couple weeks.

Libby Char The day that we were there, the hospital capacity for COVID patients was well over ninety. We asked what the capacity was to trigger another unit and they were about three patients away from that, so they were already planning to open what I think would have been the third unit for COVID because they were overflowing. We were still on the way up prior to the Fourth of July weekend, and a lot of the concern was there's already fatigue. *We're already stretched, we're three patients away from opening up a whole other unit for COVID, and they were very worried about it. When is this going to end? There's no end in sight. We're tired, we're all working overtime, and we've been doing this for months now.* There was concern about that because we were still on that upward trajectory.

You gained a lot of respect that day because you actually went and saw firsthand—that was a big deal. You let people voice what they thought and you listened to them. They felt like they were heard. That was a big deal. And you never tried to politicize that. You never made a big media deal about the fact that you had been there. You mentioned it, but you didn't try to politicize that. And they very much respected that. There really was a reason why you went there, and for the reason they were hoping it was, and so I heard back from a lot people we had seen that day. They respected you very much for that visit.

Kirk Caldwell After going to the hospital, we wrote the order again, modified the order that we initially did, and sent it to the governor. And I think the governor acted pretty quickly. Of course, people now are really upset. What they would tell me is, "You know, Mayor, the first shutdown is like you cut off someone's arm and they bled, but we stopped the bleeding. The second shutdown is we don't have as much blood anymore. You cut off our other arm. Now we're going to just die, bleed out, because we don't have enough blood. And we're bleeding again."

But I told them health and safety is more important than anything else and we can't have one without the other. At three hundred cases, we're going to hit that spike. We're going to have a thousand cases and so it needed to be done.

So after that weekend, we came back and did another stay-at-home, work-from-home order, sent it over to the governor, and he granted it.

Maui mayor Mike Victorino described how the second surge and shutdown affected Maui County.

Mike Victorino Our county is different because we have three separate islands. We had an outbreak on Lāna'i, so we immediately shut down. It was pretty easy because it's one small island with a population of about 3,300 people. However, it got more complex as we got to Maui because of the diversity and size of Maui. We shut down and we set up checkpoints to travel in and out of Hāna, and within Hāna—that helped a lot. Cases were spreading in Hāna, and for a while we had things under control. When we had the big surge in the summer, Maui was very fortunate that we didn't have really large numbers.

You folks were really catching it on O'ahu and others were having major problems so we started intercounty lockdowns. We checked everyone coming in and out of Maui County from outside of the county. It created a lot of challenges, but it also kept our case counts down. Plus, the Safe Travels was already in place for Mainland travelers. Testing was a big thing. We did an immense amount of testing during that period—May, June, July, and into August 2020 when we finally wrapped up testing. It really helped prevent spread because we were able to isolate specific areas. Harbor Lights (condominium in Kahului, Maui) had a major cluster but we could isolate, get in there, sanitize and clean, quarantine groups of people, and care for those in isolation, and we slowed it down really well.

Kirk Caldwell Hāna is a unique place. You had kind of a roadblock where people could only go to Hāna who lived in Hāna. Could you explain why you did that for that community in particular and how it worked and how it was received and how difficult was it to implement and continue to do it until it was no longer required to do it?

Mike Victorino We needed the State's approval first because Hāna Highway going in from Central Maui, Haʻikū into Hāna, is controlled by the State. The back end coming into Kula, from Kaupō and Kanaio, is controlled by the County. We were able to set up the roadblocks with the governor's approval because Hāna is such a small community. It's isolated, with very limited medical facilities, so they allowed us to do that. And it worked fairly well. We kept the case counts down, did a lot of community testing during that period of time, and we got the situation under control.

The same thing happened with Lānaʻi during their big outbreak. We shut the island down, did a lot of testing, and quickly got things under control.

Molokaʻi was a little more difficult because although we shut the island down once or twice, it was more difficult because the residents travel between Lānaʻi, Molokaʻi, and Maui for medical and business reasons, so it makes it difficult to completely shut those areas down.

Kirk Caldwell For Hāna again, because of the lack of medical facilities out in that very isolated region—I would imagine they were very appreciative that you saw it as a special place that needed to be protected. Was that the feeling of the residents out there? That you recognized that and you wanted to make sure they were not harmed in any way?

Mike Victorino Yes, they were very appreciative and it was really well received. Because it was really to protect the well-being of Hāna residents. The people on Lānaʻi felt the same way. Both communities were very appreciative of shutdowns that protected them when the case counts grew.

Kirk Caldwell You had more than two outbreaks at Maui Memorial.

There was that one early on and then I think there could have been a second one that I know you talked a lot about it. Can you describe that and how you felt and what you did to try to control it?

Mike Victorino Hawaii Healthcare Systems controls Maui Memorial. Our hospital is a division of Hawaii Healthcare Systems managed by the nonprofit Maui Health. The first outbreak was caused by the lack of PPE. The first real issue involved policies like wearing masks, not needing to wear masks, and other issues that came out during about a two-month period. Corrective measures were put in place and we were able to take care of the problem and reduce the number of cases. The spread occurred within the hospital itself.

The second surge, which was back in August/September, was really spread coming into the hospital from the community. People were getting a little nonchalant because visitors were coming back, the state had reopened, and some people felt like the pandemic was over. Which was far from the truth.

Kirk Caldwell Again, Maui Memorial is not really your *kuleana*, but I thought, of all the mayors, you took a very strong position even though it was a State responsibility. I just remember thinking you were a very strong and forceful leader demanding action to stem the spread at the hospital.

Mike Victorino They worked closely with me, and I'm very proud of the working relationship we developed there. They realized some of the early mistakes that were made and they did a great job in correcting them. We assisted by helping with their supply chain and we gave the hospital $3.8 million of our CARES Act funds to help establish another warm unit (a type of hospital unit) to separate COVID patients from others. Even with the current surge, that warm unit has been reactivated and is working pretty well. We had to be part of the solution. Not just talk about it, but do something to help them. And we did everything we could. And we still continue to support them in every way possible.

Kirk Caldwell I think, of all the mayors, you led the charge on this inter-county testing. First we stopped all travel from the continent, and then you felt O'ahu had so many cases, you asked the governor to require testing between the islands. I supported it and I was not against requiring testing. And I think it actually stemmed the spread to your county and others.

Mike Victorino When the summer surge started, the island of O'ahu was having such high numbers—O'ahu was in triple digits while most of the other counties were in single or sometimes double digits. I felt it was prudent to test people coming into Maui or to make sure they had an exemption to come for essential work. The whole plan was to prevent spread coming in from O'ahu.

We did not restrict intra-county travel between Maui County's three islands because we travel by boat or plane to get to these other parts of my county. Whereas on O'ahu or the Big Island or Kaua'i, people can drive throughout the entire county. So I didn't require testing for intra-county travel.

Maui people going to O'ahu never had to get tested, but they did have to be tested to come home.

As cases increased exponentially in August, Sherry Menor-McNamara knew that the business community faced a second shutdown but wondered if they would survive a second round. Many issues revolved around communication, or lack of it, and confusion over who had the authority to shut down the state.

Sherry Menor-McNamara (Chamber of Commerce Hawai'i) We didn't get any notice—just through media, which caused even more confusion. It would've helped to at least have gotten a heads up that you planned to shut down the state.

There was a lot of confusion about who had authority. The governor? The mayor? And what are the dynamics of the whole thing? Whose order do we follow? Initially, there was a lot of confusion and there was a feeling that communication wasn't clear.

Kirk Caldwell Libby Char said if we didn't shut down a second time we would have had a huge problem in our state. People dying in the hallways of hospitals. We could have let business stay open and we'd figure out who the bad guys were. I don't know how we'd figure that out. There are cases all over the place. Who knows where they're coming from? But we knew one thing, shutting down brought down the number of cases. It hurt business, but I don't know of a model where you stay open, wide open, in our country, in a spike, and just shutter the places where bad things were happening. Because by then it was spreading rapidly and popping up everywhere.

If we had more testing and contact tracing we could have avoided the second shutdown, and we pushed like crazy.

Sherry Menor-McNamara Businesses felt like, *We're not causing it but again we're shutting down.* There were some cases at businesses and some of them shut down on their own, like gyms, knowing that they didn't want to risk anything for their employees and customers. The other gyms did follow the health guidelines and went above and beyond. There were some that just didn't and that's where businesses felt, *Why us? We're doing everything right.* I think that was one of the biggest complaints.

When things first started opening up, we put together a small business advisory council of industries that felt that they were the most impacted—so gyms, bars, restaurants, sports, attractions, and wedding businesses—just to start to have a discussion, find solutions. You talked with them, too. They were very vocal, frustrated.

One of the ideas that came out of it that was almost finalized was the *mana* program. It's a sort of gold star program where if the business is going above and beyond, implementing everything the DOH lays out, then they can remain open in the event there was a shutdown. So DOH would be part of it. The counties would be a part of it as well, but if you have a mana seal, then that would at least provide some incentive for businesses to comply. For those who didn't comply, set up a hotline so people can call and say, "Hey, check on this restaurant," and that's when the Honolulu Liquor Commission or whatever means of enforcement will follow up. Was it the solution? I don't know, but at least it was an idea as a way to keep businesses that are following the rules open. In the end, it didn't come together.

Kirk Caldwell It still could be a good program to have. If there's a mutation and pretty soon we're not immune to the mutation, we're back to where we were. I don't think we'll shut down again, but we could, and anyone who's certified can stay open.

In the summer of 2020, prior to the second surge, Paul Yonamine was actively working on implementing a travel bubble agreement with Japan.

Paul Yonamine (Central Pacific Bank) Actually, around June or July we really had an opportunity to effect a travel bubble with Japan. We had Japan's foreign minister at that time, Toshimitsu Montegi, talking in public forums about starting travel with Hawai'i, which felt very positive. And we spent a lot of time with Mr. [Koichi] Ito, the consul general here, talking to the Hawai'i Congress Friendship Committee, which is headed by Congressman Matsuyama. All the stars were aligning, but then the State skipped a beat with the insufficient number of contact tracers it had employed and we spiked in August. The travel bubble was dead after that spike.

I know this because I spoke with the foreign ministry in Japan soon thereafter and they said they didn't want to talk about a travel bubble again. We had an opportunity to start it and lost it. Then again, Tokyo had its issues too. Its COVID rates were spiking, although with fewer fatalities. Would the travel bubble have persisted? It's hard to say. I don't want to be too punitive in my comments because, again, nobody really knew how this whole experience was going to play out. At the time, though, in June and July of 2020, we really pursued this opportunity and spent all the right time with all the right people. The work was paying off, but then when Hawai'i infections spiked we were done.

The Japanese government was even willing to carve Hawai'i out from the Mainland US and give us a different rating on COVID. It took a lot of work and I was personally very involved so I was so disappointed when it fell through. There were supposed to be two-hundred-something tracers—and there were only seventeen. I don't run the bank this way. I go and I inspect our operations and I make sure that we're compliant. When people don't spend those five minutes to do what they should overseeing others, they don't have an excuse. I was extremely upset about that experience.

Dennis Francis (Oahu Publications) The second lockdown was really ominous—kind of a ball buster. October, November, and December are big months for us and for most newspapers across the country. It's when we make a lot of our money from advertising as we head into the holidays. We were looking forward to that last quarter, and then we get locked down in August. That really threw everyone for a loop, took the wind out of our sails.

Retailers and a lot of consumers start to think, *We better hunker down for the long term*, that this could go on for a long time. When the holidays approached, they were very conservative. When I would call you, Mayor, with thoughts about some of the businesses that could reopen during that lockdown, it really wasn't from my perspective because none of those sectors were big advertisers for us. I wasn't looking at it from an economic standpoint for the newspaper. I was looking at it as just common sense for the community.

People were frustrated. They wanted to go out and do things, and I thought there had to be a better way to give some of these businesses a chance to survive and stay open until things get better. Things like allowing restaurants to do takeout and outside dining definitely helped. I thought there could have been more thought put into the car dealership restrictions since most of that business is conducted outdoors. People spend very little time inside some office closing the deal. Most of the transaction is out in the parking lot and test driving. I thought that was a little too restrictive and could have been handled better. When you're from my side, you guys in government don't necessarily feel it and touch it enough to know the difference. So I was trying to give you that touch point—that you could do something differently and make things a little better for people.

The second surge hit Hawai'i at the time of year when schools, public and private, would normally be preparing for the fall start of the school year. It became clear that this was not only not going to happen, but that there was a good chance that schools would close for the remainder of the calendar year.

Christina Kishimoto (Hawai'i DOE) We had kind of this little hui going of charter, private, public, where we would get together every other week and just have a conversation about *What are you doing? Why are you doing it?* I had much more access to information—what was happening nationally, access to the mayors, access to the governor—than they did. They wanted to know if we were willing to share with them. *Sure, just download and this is what I'm gonna do/this is why I'm doing it.* So there were some things that we did the same across public and private because of those conversations and that was helpful. It was about making sure our kids are okay.

Then we had meetings with the unions. We had more meetings than we had hours in the week. We met on a weekly basis with the unions for an entire year. And I insisted that it was all of the unions at once. HSTA, UPW, HGEA, they were all present, those are the three. I would share what decision I was making so they knew and they weren't surprised, and I would say HGEA and UPW in particular were really good about saying, "You tell us what you need from us and we will work with you." I appreciated that. If I had three unions pulling me in three directions that would have been harder.

For the teachers union, they came on strong at first saying it's not safe for any teacher to come back. And I said, "You know what? We've had food service workers, principals, my team—there are some of us who never went home and we haven't had any spread amongst us. We have a safety protocol in place." That's the other thing that I think is a big check mark for DOE—none of us got sick off of serving our community.

Soon as vaccines were available, we were the first in line. We're interacting with a lot of people. We can't get sick and go spread it. So we wanted to make sure we held to our responsibility.

But at first, HSTA said no teacher was safe. And I said, "No, this is not just about teachers vs. anyone else. What I have—I have a group of kids in crisis, I have a group of kids that are special ed, I have kids who can't interact with technology because of their special needs so those teachers have to come back unless you're telling me that I'm shutting the system down for them. And if I'm shutting it down for them, by federal law I have to shut it down for every child. So you're telling me we're shutting down the school system, and if you're going to refuse to come to work, then I'm going to refuse to pay. We're not paying salaries then. We're going to shut down officially. We're going to save on salaries until we open up and then we'll start paying again." Well that changed the conversation at the table. But that was the reality. I can't pay folks for not working. I can't do that and I also can't just tell kids that we're not available to teach you.

On prioritization, I think we all came to consensus quickly, like special ed kids that can't learn online. We have special ed kids that can learn online and did great. Our English language learners who had huge impediments with the English language. We can't put them on a computer. We didn't have enough language experts. And our students in crisis who didn't have the social network at home—they were going to be in potential danger at home. There were parents who said, "I'm an emergency worker. I have no one at home and I have a first grader. What do I do with my child? I can't leave my child alone." So we made sure we kept asking parents, "Who's at home? Do you have an adult at home?" Constantly checking in. And I'm sure that there are children that stayed home all alone, but we kept checking because my biggest fear during this time period was a child getting hurt at home. Thankfully, we have not heard of any and hopefully we won't learn that some child did get hurt.

Suicide was the other thing. We had surveys that went out to kids that informed us there was a huge spike in the number of kids that said they felt sad and alone. Those are the ones that we were trying to bring back as quickly as possible. This included creating rooms where they could bring their technology and an adult would be supervising—it didn't need to be a teacher, we just didn't want that child alone. We made the decision that they would come into what we call learning hubs, digital hubs where they could get connectivity.

It was a lot of moving parts at once.

Kirk Caldwell Then you had the graduations. Chief Ballard was pretty hard-assed about things, but we listened to her and respected her. She is the chief of police. But you had kids who were looking forward to proms, junior prom, senior prom, graduation, all these major events we remember in our lives that they don't get to have and they're sad and depressed. You're dealing with parents and kids, and then the politicians in each county and the State making decisions, and the chiefs.

Christina Kishimoto So at the end of that first year, it was the first quarter that we shut down, that was just a time period of confusion for everyone. I had mayors calling me, saying, "I want to make this decision for my county. I can't do that. That is so different from your decision." So I tried as hard as possible to create the collaboration around reducing confusion for kids and families. That was the important thing. Just having some consistency.

Kirk Caldwell We said no to you at the end of the day on some things. You wanted graduations.

Christina Kishimoto There were a couple things that some of our high schools wanted that Honolulu County said no to, but then all the counties had some nuanced differences.

Kirk Caldwell But you never threw us under the bus. I never heard anyone say, "Yeah, the superintendent says she wanted to do it but the mayor said no at the county." I never heard that.

Christina Kishimoto I think I recognized that it was just a confusing time. It was hard to blame anyone for the fact that everyone was trying to make the best decision. And we talked a lot about that as a team. We kept saying, "Look, everyone's trying to do good. No one's trying to create chaos." But at the same time, how do you tell a county mayor you made the wrong decision—it was your fault? That doesn't make sense either, right?

Kirk Caldwell Another thing is sports. We were pretty tough on sports, Oʻahu—I don't know about the other islands, but you've got important rivalries. How did you deal with that? You've got a whole bunch of parents saying, "Why can't we practice outside? You can have five in a restaurant, but you can't have a team on the field?"

Christina Kishimoto I never got any comment that said, "What's the mayor doing?" For me it was always like, "What are you doing?" I would get blamed for a decision that wasn't necessarily a decision from me. I was constantly trying to say that all decision makers are trying to make the best decisions right now; there's so much we don't know about this virus.

David Lassner (University of Hawaiʻi) Like most organizations, we kept hoping for a return to normalcy. Every time we thought we'd be able to return to in-person presence we were hit by another surge, first Delta and then Omicron. The major lesson we learned was the importance of staying flexible. While our students and faculty and staff all wanted certainty, the reality is that decisions needed to be responsive to whatever wrinkles COVID threw at us and those have just not been predictable.

On the Big Island, Harry Kim was becoming frustrated working with the federal, state, and the private sectors encompassing a comprehensive plan in responding to the virus.

Harry Kim (Mayor of Hawaiʻi County) My major difference with policy makers on the federal and the state level is on the outlook of our responses. I have said this to the governor and all the mayors, that my emphasis and outlook are based on an operational outlook and not just principles and policies. This was always the problem because of my background on operations.

By this time, Dr. Jonathan Dworkin had moved to Hawaiʻi Island and began working at the Queen's North Hawai'i facility in Waimea. He was in touch with Mayor Kim on COVID matters on the Big Island, and he continued to be part of Mayor Caldwell's advisory panel in Honolulu on the weekly video conference meetings.

Jonathan Dworkin (Queen's Health System) Since the vaccine's come out, you've got a really good new tool to change the shape of things, but in 2020 it was, "Can you identify where the virus is? Can you contact trace in a timely way? Can you separate infected from uninfected, and either help them quarantine at home or support them at a centralized quarantine location?" Those were sort of the key tools and one of the debates that played out that I think was an academic debate that people were really slow to adjust on: Is this traditional model of testing a doctor-ordered test? Who interprets the test?

And if I order a test and it comes back negative, I get this kind of academic scolding like, "Why are you wasting resources driving up the cost of healthcare?" And there's some validity to this because you don't want to go to the kind of doctor who orders a bunch of unnecessary tests.

So one of the arguments I was having especially early on at Queen's was to try to get them out of this one-test-per-doctor way of thinking. And I don't think the DOH ever left that paradigm. I think they were stuck in that 2019 paradigm throughout the entire course. It wasn't until the leadership change did they ever shift out of it. Queen's did shift out of it eventually, but it took a few weeks to get them to divorce themselves from the DOH approach and it's hard because it's habit shifting. You're basically telling a bunch of doctors, "This isn't about you. Get out of the way. This is about testing and scale and likewise connecting that to the other services you know as well as I do at this point. The contact tracing, the isolation, the quarantine, the wraparound care." And if you looked around for successful models, that's what you saw in all the successful models.

One of the things you had to do in order to be able to embrace this is first you had to stop listening to the DOH and the CDC, which was hard for a lot of people. And then you had to look around the world and see what places were doing well with coronavirus. You're looking at places like Taiwan and Korea and New Zealand. And okay, what are they doing? They have border control, they do test, trace, isolate very aggressively. They have homegrown testing that they've supported as part of their own biotech industries, and they're sort of charting their own course. I was pushing for those things because that's what I saw working in other parts of the world and there were some very smart people. This wasn't just coming into my own head. There were some very smart people on the Mainland—people like Trevor Bedford at University of Washington, Michael Mina at Harvard School of Public Health. Some very bright academics on the Mainland were saying the same thing, and I was essentially reading their stuff and saying it here. But the key step was to sort of disrupt the traditional approach towards testing and move away from this model of everything is about the individual patient/doctor encounter. And what you're trying to move towards is the public health strategy to try to control sort of a fire.

Kirk Caldwell In a pandemic, the usual rules don't apply. We're in a pandemic but they're applying the same rules, so you saw that within your own organization, within doctors that you know. I get so upset with the DOH but I wonder if health departments are not set up to deal with pandemics?

Jonathan Dworkin I think there was a cultural adjustment and different people made the adjustments at different speeds. But I think you're absolutely right. What does the DOH do well? I think their TB control branch is a good branch. TB is a kind of slow-moving infection; their slow speed doesn't hurt them much with TB and they've been doing it for a hundred years. There's stuff that they've been doing for a hundred years—venereal diseases, tuberculosis—unsurprisingly, they're better at those things.

So the pandemic was just much more fast moving and they needed to be able to adjust. But they had trouble culturally adjusting. A lot of health departments, the people who staff them, they're trained in CDC epi courses. So they're very CDC-centric. If the CDC is moving quickly, they're more likely to move quickly. If the CDC is in chaos, then you've got fifty state health departments that are likely to be in chaos.

The places that succeeded, I think, for example on Kaua'i, Janet Berreman pretty early on started charting her own course. And the mayor there was bright and listened to her. The two of them formed a good working relationship with each other. So it wasn't like everyplace. Still, there were individual officers. On the Big Island, when I got over here, I had a meeting with Harry Kim, and the district health officer on the Big Island was right next to him. And there was a completely coordinated effort. So Harry Kim was kind of an eccentric guy, but one thing that I noticed right away was that he had a good relationship with the DOH, at least on the island here, and they were willing to do stuff for him.

I think on O'ahu you suffered from being next to DOH central. And you had all the dysfunction of DOH central, but on some of the neighboring islands they were a little bit more innovative. I don't know about other states but I do remember hearing very similar stories. I went to Brown. My colleagues at Brown were incensed with the dysfunction of the Rhode Island Department of Health. They had a massive epidemic there and they were going at this very plodding course. I think it needs to be reformed. One of the points David Derauf has made to me—you should ask him about this because he has more connections within the public health community in general—was that there was a lot of brain drain at the CDC prior to the pandemic. Even prior to Trump, going all the way back to Ebola, but I think it accelerated under Trump. So they didn't necessarily have the middle tier. They had extremely high-quality middle-tier people that is the professional core of that organization. A lot of them moved on to other jobs. And you were left with a lot of political appointees and people who just wanted things to be as normal as possible and weren't as comfortable rocking the boat.

Perhaps the most disadvantaged community on O'ahu in terms of understanding what was happening with COVID and then adapting their lives in order to stay healthy was the Pacific Islander community. The infection rate among this community was the highest in the state due to many factors including language and cultural barriers, and immensely crowded living conditions. Dr. David Derauf, Kōkua Kalihi Valley, was a critical advocate for Pacific Islanders and other disadvantaged groups.

David Derauf I think it was important to do it [lockdown] right at the beginning, because we didn't know enough, we didn't know how to treat the disease, all the initial focus seemed to be on using ventilators and no focus on good ventilation, etc.

You were one of the few people I remember helping to push for isolation quarters to be made available early on. DOH was moving more slowly on that and the City did come through on support in this and other key areas.

Kirk Caldwell Can we talk a little bit about the Pacific Islanders? I don't think I effectively interfaced with the Pacific Islanders before the pandemic, during the pandemic, or after. Some, but there was so much work that needed to be done. So we had these shutdowns, two of them. You've got the Pacific Islanders who were basically the backbone of all the dirtiest, lowest-paying work, whether the back of restaurants, care homes, hospitals. For the most part, a lot of them still had to go to work. So they hear about these shutdowns. You say government doesn't really talk to them, they don't know about it, they hear about it through their church or however they hear it. How are they feeling? Are they afraid? They're thinking, *How am I going to pay my rent? Am I going to work? What if I get sick?* They're worried too.

David Derauf My very first patient with COVID was a thirty-eight-year-old woman. I called her up and said, "Your test came back positive." Silence. And I had known her; she'd been my patient. Chuukese. We didn't have a strong relationship, but we had a strong beginning to a relationship already. I said, "We need to ask you to isolate yourself. What's your living circumstances like?" "Well, there's eight of us in a two-bedroom." "Is there a way you can have a room to yourself?" Hard. "You can't go to work tomorrow. You must stay home from work." She said, "I'm the only one in the house with an income right now. What happens to us if I don't go to work?"

Fortunately, her only symptom was a headache. A bad headache. "But you can't go to work tomorrow. You're going to infect your coworkers." She was in fast food. "Dr. Derauf, if I don't pay the rent, where do you think we're going to be?" That was my first eye-opener. *The easy part of this is to test you. Now I have got the hard part, which is what are we going to do for you? How are we going to support you?*

So we started taking that seriously—processing food baskets with rice, medicine, masks, hand sanitizer, canned goods—because, again, DOH got around to them but it wasn't for two or three days to get it lined up. So if we could cover those first few days it would help.

I did our death review three weeks ago (summer 2021) for Kōkua Kalihi Valley. It's very interesting to look and see. We had about eight hundred cases of COVID that we had managed by then. We're not far off the state average for mortality. Hawai'i's had about 1.3% case fatality rate at that time. Kōkua Kalihi Valley, I think we were at about 1.6% case fatality rate. Which given the high-risk community we serve, to me that tells you supporting people, knocking on doors, phoning, or Zooming in to check in on them daily, giving them fresh food, getting them into isolation if they needed to be there—all that made a huge difference in people's lives.

There are a few things that might have compounded the experience in our community. For example, funeral ceremonies. They're important for all of us, any culture, but in the Chuukese community that is considered the glue that holds the community together. The funeral. It is as central a part of their culture as anything. So suddenly we told them, "Sorry, you can't gather at a funeral."

People are like, "You're going to ruin our culture. We are not who we are if we don't do funerals." So there's one I can't wrap my mind around again, because how do we do it safely and how do we recognize for them there are worse things than dying and one of them is to not honor your ancestors?

The third time I got really scared during the pandemic was when someone had died. It was a funeral of a prominent person in the Pacific Islander community, and I knew a lot of people would be coming into town to attend. They came from the West Coast, Vegas, Seattle, LA, and some of the staff said, "Dr. Derauf, I have to put up some of these people who came for the funeral. My house isn't safe."

Kirk Caldwell Are they in a worse place or a better place now? And why?

David Derauf Oh, a much better place. The leadership in the community really did stand up. A lot of times the messages that I was bringing to our mayors meeting was what I had learned by listening to some of these ministers. One man took me to task. We have a weekly meeting. Every Tuesday night we meet with a group of ministers. A Zoom. And early on, June/July of last year, one of the ministers said point-blank, "Dr. Derauf, I walk into your testing clinic tomorrow morning, I test positive. What are you going to do? You sending me home? I live with a bunch of sick people you know. You going to send me home? I'm not coming in to get tested until you can tell me what you're going to do. What's the next step?"

I knew then we had to commit. Our goal was, within four hours, we're going to have you placed in an isolation facility. We're going to keep you here, we're going to bring you food, we're going to use those hours to educate you about this illness, and we're going to have your trust that you're going to tell your family to come in and get tested because we're going to take care of you. If we tell them otherwise—"Just come in and get tested and you're on your own," which is what happened to most to people in the US, even to this day we're still doing that—we're not really helping them.

Kirk Caldwell Well, think about it. Yesterday, 655 people were told you're positive. What happened to those 655 people? They went home? Who knows, they could have even gone in to work. If I had tested positive and I didn't tell you, you wouldn't know.

David Derauf We know many went into work, we know many of them live in crowded quarters, we know that most of them aren't given any message about what you can do proactively at home. Nutritional support, rest, fresh air, daily check-ins with your doctor—almost none of them get that. Eighteen months into this thing, and for many people with COVID we're still at a point where we're telling them, "Oh, you're positive. Go home and if you get worse go to the ER."

Jonathan Dworkin (Queen's Health System) I have a question about the police, Mayor. This is something that I've always been curious about. Because in my mind, the whole thing with the beaches, I thought that the best thing for them to have done would have been to basically use crowd sizes to determine police behavior. We never really wanted to discourage people from going outside but we ended up having to do that because they said either it's open or closed. And I'm wondering if there was something going on in the background there. Were they angry about what had happened with the Black Lives Matter protests? Were they refusing to cooperate in a way they could have? Because one thing I noticed when I got over here was that it seemed like the relationship between county and police was a little less contentious.

Now it's true they weren't asking the police to do very much in terms of crowd control. But I always wondered afterwards. I wasn't privy to your internal conversations with police, but was there something there? Were they afraid they were going to be called racist if they broke up a big Polynesian beach gathering? What was their actual concern?

Kirk Caldwell Well, I think part of it is could they actually break up a large Polynesian beach gathering without incredible show of force? The first time we opened up pretty quickly. Every Saturday and Sunday our beaches around the island including Waikīkī looked like the Fourth of July. All local people. I told my wife, "You gotta come down. You gotta see this. It's all local people. There's not one tourist." And I do think that surge that we saw in July and August came partly from that. Not actually because they were close together, hanging out all day at the beach, but they went home and stayed close together afterwards. Everyone got lax. *It's okay. Hey, we were at the beach all day. Let's go hang out at grandma's house, uncle's house, auntie's house.* And so I think a lot of that spread, with no proof, came from there.

When it really got out of hand, I did ask the chief if they could enforce. She said, "It's too hard at this point. It's way out of control. We need a relationship with this community after the pandemic. And if we're out there trying to do this, when it's done, we'll have no relationship with the community and we do need that relationship." And I said, "Fair enough."

But when we locked down the second time, I did go to her and said, "We're going to open up again," and to your point, it was her recommendation—and we may put this in the law, our order when we open—was that you could have small gatherings but anything over ten with a tent, you needed a permit from the Department of Parks and Recreation. So they did. So that came out first. She said, "We will enforce if we have these requirements so we can at least go in quickly when a tent pops up and say, 'Do you have your permit?' and 'Only ten.'" She even said how far apart the tents had to be because she didn't want to pore over large multigenerational families having multiple tents. And they did enforce the second time, as you may recall. They did over sixty thousand citations, most of them were thrown out—fifty-eight thousand were thrown out. We ended up offering the state court system a couple million dollars of our CARES money to process a lot of these. But she actually did step up.

And she got beat up for it. But that's how I see it. The first time, they weren't ready for the surge and by the time all this happened it was too hard to clamp it down. The second time, we realized this could occur again, but we were ready for it, and I think we controlled it a lot better.

She said, "If we're going to do this on tents, we're going to do it on everything. Anyone who goes into a park not to swim, we're gonna cite 'em." She cited the surgeon general of the United States. I was told to say, "Tell them not to do anything." But I said, "Guys, I told the chief I'm going to back her up. Everyone who gets a citation, I'm not going to interfere. It's the court that can decide."

Jonathan Dworkin That was Jerome Adams. When did that happen? That was like in August or something like that? That was around the time of the second shutdown.

Kirk Caldwell Yeah, the second shutdown, because we were doing badly. We had 355 cases in a day for a population of a million. What happened was Dr. Deborah Birx (White House COVID-19 response coordinator)—the one who wore the scarf and stood next to Trump and sometimes looked embarrassed by what he was saying—she called me up and said, "Mayor, I used to work at Tripler and we're concerned about your city. What can we do to help?" I said, "I want remdesivir," more of that, and I said we need more testing.

She said, "We can help you with that. The surgeon general is going to call you about surge testing." And then he called me. I was shocked that he actually called and he said, "I wanna do it. I'm going to come out."

The other thing, I visited Queen's on Statehood Day in August at your request and suggestion, which led to my coming back and saying we're going to do a second stay-at-home, work-from-home order.

Jonathan Dworkin I noticed afterwards you came out and you seemed to really have a firm sense of direction. And then the order came the next week, and then we were talking about the DOH. You didn't stop with the order. You managed to get the leadership at the DOH changed.

Kirk Caldwell It took a week because partly we prepared the order quickly. We just took our old order and modified it, but convincing the governor and Bruce Anderson to do this was really hard. When I finally got their agreement to do it, we were sitting in the governor's cabinet room—that big room next to his office—and we're saying, *Okay, the governor's going to go out and say this. He's going to support the City and County of Honolulu. Mayor, you're going to do this. Bruce you're going to do this.* And Bruce goes, "Well I don't agree with this." Now this is after we all agreed we're going to do it. Literally five minutes, straighten your hair, take your pen out of your pocket, tuck in your shirt, and now he's saying he's having second thoughts.

I slammed my hand on the table. I stood up and said, "I'm out of here. I'm gone. Goodbye. Really, Governor? After a week of discussing it, we all agreed, and now we're going to go out and implement, we're crawling out of the foxhole, and one of the guys is saying I'm not going with you. The director of the DOH! This is ridiculous!"

Then Bruce said okay. He said, "No, I'll say I support it." But I'm thinking at this point, *This guy's gotta go. Gotta go.*

At the end of August, Honolulu was in the second lockdown, and the mayor asked the City's Corporation Counsel to work with the state attorneys and the DOH to develop a new system that would enable O'ahu to reopen, when the time was right, in a more systematic way.

Another significant change was that on August 31, 2020, the director of health, Bruce Anderson, resigned his position.

David Ige (Governor of Hawai'i) I have always believed, as governor, that I wanted to hire leaders, and I wanted them to be empowered to run their agencies. I served in the legislature a long time. I saw how governors would hire directors and they wouldn't be authorized to make any decisions. In building the cabinet, I made it clear that I expected directors to lead. And then obviously I think that most leaders are aware that there are some decisions that they can make and it's more administrative, and then there are some decisions that clearly have to come back to me as governor. It's about the relationship that you have with the individual directors.

My concern at that point: We're in the middle of a pandemic, at what point do you change leadership? I had conversations with both Bruce Anderson and Sarah Park and I shared a lot of their beliefs about what things should and shouldn't be happening in response to the pandemic.

It became obvious that we would need to make a change, but to have a leadership change in the middle of a public health emergency is not the best time to be able to do that. And certainly a big concern of mine was how the agency would respond and what it would mean from the public health perspective about how or who would be making decisions.

Bruce came to talk to me. He told me that he was becoming a distraction and that he would be retiring. I expressed my appreciation and asked for time to figure out a transition to new leadership because "I can't have you retire without having somebody in place to lead DOH, especially in the middle of a health emergency."

I had actually recruited Libby Char very heavily when I was formulating my second cabinet. I had offered her the position and in the end she declined when we were putting that cabinet together.

I talked with Libby again—I had actually talked to several people about serving as director once Bruce told me that he would step aside. We had to make sure that we had someone to lead the agency. Finally, Libby agreed to do it. So we proceeded to make the change in a way that would not be disruptive and create a leadership vacuum. ✻

CHAPTER 5

Tiers and Fears

Over the Labor Day weekend of 2020, a team of attorneys and administrators representing the governor and Honolulu's mayor hunkered down to create a tier system that would allow O'ahu to open up in a measured and systematic way. It was clear that decisions on what to open and when to open needed more structure and more transparency. While not perfect, it allowed residents and businesses to better understand what needed to happen before reaching a specific tier, and perhaps community behavior would then be modified by the "carrot" of reaching the criteria. Bad numbers, however, meant the possibility of reverting back to a more closed tier. The reactions from the community were both positive and negative. And even if one did not agree with the criteria to reach the next tier—for example, the differing markers for restaurants and bars were a heated topic—the daily COVID numbers were closely tracked, and the number of cases and the positivity rate became part of the public conversation. Libby Char was part of that team.

Libby Char (Hawai'i DOH) The City creating the tier system, when nobody else really had, was one of the most stabilizing forces. Contact tracing was ongoing and by creating the tier system, that put a little bit of structure to help the public realize how significant it was that there were rules in place, and once people understood what the rules were, that helped to kind of calm everybody down.

People were still very anxious about it, but there was a structure there and people could understand what the rules were. They didn't like them necessarily, but I think it was a tremendously stabilizing action.

The other thing was when we amended the tier system and we were saying, "Don't open the restaurants yet," and you opened the restaurants, you said up front, very publicly, in a press conference that the public health and medical people were advising against it, but you were going to do it anyway and that you took responsibility for it.

The public health folks, the people that worked on the tier system, a lot of people in the medical community really respected you for that. For doing what you thought had to be done, but very publicly saying this is what medical recommends, you were going to do something different and that you owned it. Because sometimes I think there's a feeling from the medical side that had you done that and not publicly said that, that the message is that the medical community condones that. You allowed the medical and public health guidance to be documented that that was their position and that you were taking responsibility for not specifically following it.

Kirk Caldwell The other thing that I appreciated is when Sarah Kemble (the DOH epidemiologist) talked about it at the press conference and explained why the DOH team and others didn't think restaurants should open to other than takeout. I thought it was important for the public to know, for those who are listening to the health side, so that they have more information to decide whether they're going to go to a restaurant, and that's important information. I was concerned for all those people who are employed in the restaurant business. Restaurants are a major sector of our economy on Oʻahu, but I didn't want to imply that there's no risk. Hearing from a DOH doctor on whether it is safe to eat in a restaurant at that point in time is important information for the public to take into consideration. You can go, but you may not want to.

So can we talk a little bit about the tier system and your role in developing the tiers and metrics? You had a key role in this intense, multiday marathon.

Libby Char We did several long days. We got together as a city and put something together. I think we did a pretty good job with it. We hammered out a lot of the framework and then either the following week or a couple weeks later a team from the State joined and we worked on it together. That was really important because everybody's input was heard and it was so helpful to have the AG [attorney general] on the call as well as the state epidemiologist, other public health physicians as well as the City and County emergency management and legal teams. It allowed us to address issues, discuss them, and come to a common agreement right up front. And we could hear arguments from the AG that we would not otherwise have thought of, legal considerations, and so it was really helpful because at the end I think we came to a good agreement.

The attorney general was in the meetings all weekend as was I, Krishna Jayaram, Sarah Kemble, Janet Berreman, Hiro Toiya, Paul Aoki, Gabe Provenza, Ernest Nomura, Kurt Nakamatsu, and I think Ken Hara was there too. There were a lot of people putting a lot of thought and goodwill into this to come up with a good product, and I know a lot of people want to get rid of it now. I think some of them really didn't have to live through the really high case counts, so the context isn't there for them. We know so much more about COVID now. The virus has changed. We know how it works, we have some other treatment for it, so it's appropriate to amend the way we respond to it, but I think to not understand where it came from and want to get rid of everything would be a disservice to the community. Because again, then we'd have no rules, there would be no framework, and people would just be wondering.

Chris Benjamin, Alexander & Baldwin, contacted the mayor about the tier system with concerns. As representative of and landlord for a variety of small businesses, he saw how difficult it was going to be for O'ahu to move quickly through the tiers and he wanted to discuss other strategies.

Chris Benjamin It was later when you set the criteria for the number of cases and all that. And the main reason that I was calling you and trying to get involved is I was very concerned about what would happen to the restaurants if they weren't in the first tier. I was not aware of regular dine-in restaurants being the source of a lot of spread, and if they were not in that first tier, it was going to be at least another month before they could open up, and from having worked with a lot of our tenants, I knew that could be an existential event for them. That's why I wanted to try to present information to you that would frankly counter some of what you were hearing from the healthcare professionals about both the business imperative but also the safety of having restaurants and social distancing.

And that's where Mark Mugiishi was very helpful. Jason Higa, Greg Maples (from Hawai'i Restaurant Association), and of course Tina Yamaki provided some perspective. I gave you a lot of credit for being willing to have that call and consider that because I know that you were getting a lot of pressure from the healthcare folks to take a more rigid stance. And I thought it was very good the way you balanced it and agreed to let the restaurants open. I am absolutely convinced there are a lot of restaurants that exist today that would not exist if they had had to wait another month or two to open up.

Kirk Caldwell We had to get the approval of the governor who is very conservative, and the DOH was advising against it, including Janet Berreman and Sarah Kemble. They didn't want restaurants open in the first tier. In fact, the governor called me up and said, "I'm not going to let your order go into place with this in there." And then we circled back and he said, "I'll reconsider if you make it clear to everybody that this is against the advice of our DOH and your medical panel." I said not only will I do that, but I'll also invite them to my press conference and they can say it themselves. And I'll say, despite what they advise, that I'm allowing restaurants to reopen in tier 1. It could be a risk, but based on the fact that, for O'ahu only, restaurants before COVID generated approximately $1.9 billion in revenue and employed fifty-nine thousand people. In fact, they employed more people than the visitor industry, but a lot of restaurants are serving the visitor industry, and so the governor approved O'ahu's tier order. You were helpful in getting this accomplished.

Chris Benjamin Your earlier comments about Duane Kurisu (Hawai'i Executive Collaborative) and the value of having the multi-industry perspective and the industry private/public perspective is helpful, and it's something we try to do a lot of in Hawai'i, but it doesn't always work. I've always made it very clear that I am not in any way a COVID denier, I'm not reckless with health—I sent my employees home right away, but you also have to take calculated risks and you have to look at the data and I think the fact that you were willing to look at it and say, "Look, I don't think restaurants are the problem. Let's try it. And obviously if you have a bunch of spreader events in restaurants you can modify it. But let's give it a shot."

Kirk Caldwell So, on retail. You have not just restaurants but many different shopping centers, both neighborhood ones and larger ones. I think we talked about retail at some point, When is retail going to open? Do you have any thoughts on that?

Chris Benjamin The main thing I remember thinking was the fact that so many people were in Costco and Foodland and Safeway and Target for those months without face masks and without really any precautions, and there wasn't a huge surge. We had for a while, in May, very few cases. To me, that said retail was safe. And so, I remember thinking that we have proof that retail is safe and therefore being a little bit anxious to get it open again. I think Tina Yamaki felt the same way. Because if you can have all those people going into Foodland with no restrictions—later in the summer there were restrictions on how many people could be in the store, with a face mask, but back in May there was none of that. If you're an essential retailer you can be open. And the fact there were no cases being spread at that point in that setting, to me, said that retail could be safe. You're not there for prolonged periods, and you put a mask on. So I do remember feeling that we should be opening up retail, but I don't remember having the same sort of desperation that I had with restaurants. I really felt like restaurants, it was truly an existential issue for them. Plus, I think you were already moving towards opening the retail anyway. Really, the one that was in doubt was the restaurants. That's why I remember being more focused on that.

Sadly, a lot of our problems with surges were because of unsafe individual choices and actions. When we had to shut down again in August, to me, a lot of that was because people weren't being safe. I remember texting you on Memorial Day 2020 when I went to Kaimana Beach and saw how people were acting. I remember thinking, *We are in trouble.* And it continued through the summer. But what frustrated me was that people just wouldn't use common sense. Here, people's lives and businesses are at stake, yet people weren't willing to forgo a beach party. That was kind of my biggest feeling. I did not fault you or anyone for reinstating restrictions. I think it had to be done. What I did think was important though, once we had been through that open and close again, was that it was imperative that we get it right the next time and not open too quickly only to have to shut down again. That's where the tiers and the metrics were really important.

The biggest problem I had with the tier system, and I told you this, was that your tier system had an expectation that as we went through the tiers the cases would go down. My argument always was that as long as we keep the cases the same but at a sustainable level we can keep moving through the tiers.

And so, if you say we're going to do this tier for thirty days and if we don't go up, then we'll try the next tier. Rather than requiring that the cases actually come down as you open up, I always felt we should just focus on keeping cases at a sustainable level, and if we can stay at that sustainable level, fine. If the cases go up, then we'll move back.

Kirk Caldwell It's a fair point to make. Even then I found it had merit.

Chris Benjamin Your question to me was "If we don't have a lower threshold how will we know if this tier that we're in worked?" And my argument was as long as cases weren't going up, it's working. Right now, we have cases at a level that never would have been allowed in your original tier 4.

Kirk Caldwell We had two days over the weekend of over a hundred cases.

Chris Benjamin But we had very few hospitalizations. That was the other thing we talked about. What are the right criteria? Is it positivity rate? Is it cases? Is it hospitalizations? I don't know if we ever really resolved that. But Mark Mugiishi had his views, and Ray Vara had his views.

Kirk Caldwell I do think that with the vaccine rollout, which was not in place at the time the tier system was developed, you definitely could look at hospitalizations as a metric. But without the vaccinations being in place, it's a following trend. By the time you have a problem in the hospitals, you have a problem that's going to get worse. With the vaccines, I think you're right. And by the way, I do think that living with a certain number of cases, whatever that is, has to be reflective of the needs of our healthcare system. It's something we're going to have to do for a long time to come.

Chris Benjamin I would never in a hundred years say that it's worth 515 people dying so that we can do this, but the thing is I don't think that those 515 people died because stores were open. I think most of those people have died, unfortunately, because people didn't really exercise caution. They didn't wear masks, they had parties, they traveled when they shouldn't, they refused to get the vaccine—whatever it is. I think the lack of personal responsibility is more to blame for some of the health outcomes we've had than the policies have been. Generally, I think Hawai'i, as we all know, has been one of the most prudent and conservative places, yet still 515 people sadly are dead.

Kirk Caldwell I do believe the actions we took reduced that number, but I also think we could have kept it even lower if we had a more vigorous rollout of widespread testing, contact tracing, and sufficient isolation facilities early on. There's always that looking backwards.

The success of the tier system relied on messaging. It relied on everyone in the community receiving information on what was open, what was closed, and why. People's everyday lives were impacted, essentially governed, by the tiers. The Hawai'i State Department of Transportation agreed to dedicate highway electronic signage on daily case counts and positivity rates. Both the State and City spent millions of dollars on public messaging campaigns for television, radio, print, advertising walls and kiosks in shopping malls, and social media. And the state's largest newspaper publisher agreed to print the tier information and daily case counts on the front page.

Dennis Francis (Oahu Publications) Well, it made sense. As for the tier system, one of my long-standing pandemic suggestions was don't keep people in the dark on what the measuring stick is. I said put something out there so that people know that we're getting better, or not even close, or we're going to slide back into a dark hole pretty soon with these kinds of numbers. Let people know what numbers you're looking at and how you make judgements because most people will buy into it when you give them the information on what you're measuring. That's what I think the tier system did.

It made it more clear and had all the categories. It's never going to be perfect. There's never going to be a perfect system. You can make a lot of progress by getting it mostly right. So I thought that was good. And I thought that the best way for us to communicate that and show the importance of it was to have it on the front page. When you called and asked about it, that wasn't even a question. I thought it should be on the front page. The readers paid attention to it because there were always a lot of comments on it, and we would get calls if there was a discrepancy between the DOH's numbers and your numbers. *Why do you have what's on the front page and Mayor Caldwell says it's this? Which one is it?* It's because we were getting it from two different sources, so we ironed all that out, but ultimately it told us that this information was important to people, and we were right to put it on the front page.

Kirk Caldwell Do you think your paper was different from papers on the continent? Is it because we are more of a community? Do you think other papers in other states would have done what you did? Working with government and using valuable space to share information?

Dennis Francis Probably not. I think our community's a little different given that there are not a lot of newspapers our size that have a top executive who has been there a long time. Over the last decade, a lot of those people have changed out every year or two; it's somebody from another place. A Florida person is now in charge of Ohio, or an Ohio person oversees Nebraska. They're not part of that community. I've been here over thirty years, in one capacity or another. Because this is a unique place, I have long-term relationships with lots of people, including politicians. I have the ability to talk to you directly. A lot of people don't. So I took advantage of that.

The tier system essentially dictated what businesses could open, what activities could take place, and how many people could be served or could participate at any given time, depending on the tier in effect. Sherry Menor-McNamara of the Chamber of Commerce Hawai'i, had the difficult job of advocating for Hawai'i businesses, large and small, and at the same time, cooperating and brainstorming with government to keep health and safety at the forefront. The federal government in 2020 provided stimulus funding for states to help economic recovery, and because of Honolulu's size and population, the share for O'ahu came directly to the City and County, which provided about $150 million for a business program. Gary Kurokawa, the mayor's chief of staff, spearheaded that effort.

Gary Kurokawa We took money away from other programs to fund the business program. Another $50 million, I think.

Sherry Menor-McNamara That's a challenge, right? Because not everyone can qualify. Unless you give it to everybody, then it's an issue, in whatever amount. When you put thresholds, you start hearing, "How come my business does not qualify? I'm a local business. I just have fifty-one employees."

Gary Kurokawa It was a brick-and-mortar thing.

Kirk Caldwell We were trying to give to the brick-and-mortar businesses first because they are paying rent as opposed to working out of your house.

Sherry Menor-McNamara We heard a lot of criticism from home-based businesses.

Gary Kurokawa Almost every realtor. Some lawyers.

Sherry Menor-McNamara Handy men. Photographers. The wedding industry. Because they couldn't work. The bulk of the wedding industry have home-based businesses, yet they lost everything. They couldn't have any income, so I think they felt they were one of the hardest hit industries and they didn't get a fair share of it.

Kirk Caldwell If we had had more money, we would have opened it up to businesses operating out of their owners' residences. It just meant the brick-and-mortar businesses would get a less significant amount of money, and then everyone suffers. Everyone gets some, but it's not enough to make a meaningful difference.

Sherry Menor-McNamara Yeah, it's a tough call. The rent program definitely helped many businesses. We appreciate the recognition of that by putting more monies into the grant program.

Zippy's quickly surfaced as a leader in the restaurant industry. There were many factors that enabled them to weather the storm, perhaps easier than other restaurants, including the diversity of their services, their use of technology, and the number of locations around the island. Like all businesses though, the greatest struggle was how to keep the workforce employed during the recovery.

Paul Yokota (Zippy's) Initially, we had to place a large number of employees on furlough, not knowing how long the pandemic would last. When it became clear that large events would not be allowed for a lengthy period, operations like the Pomaikaʻi Ballrooms were closed and those employees were unfortunately laid off. During the pandemic, we also closed Zippy's Pearlridge and Zippy's Waimalu. As the pandemic impacts continued and sales remain depressed, we had to make some difficult decisions on our staffing. Some employees chose to retire, some employees chose not to work due to COVID concerns, and we simply had no employment opportunity for others. In the end, the total number of employees decreased by 25 percent.

Georgette Deemer I know that some of the other businesses that we've talked to, they were able to have employees work from home. But in your case, that's not possible.

Paul Yokota Yes, our restaurant employees could not work from home. However, quite a few employees on the administrative side were able to work from home, including marketing, technology, accounting, human resources, and purchasing.

Jason Higa (Zippy's) Georgette, we're so far from where we hope to be because the dine-in is still at 50 percent capacity. If you also look at our operating hours, we're closing at midnight when we used to be open twenty-four hours at many of our locations. Thus, we lost quite a bit of sales potential, and as Paul mentioned, we're at 75 percent of our pre-pandemic workforce. We are far from where we hope to be.

Paul Yokota As our restaurant operations adjusted, we made corresponding adjustments to our production as well. The operating hours and labor at our central kitchen and our central bakery production plant were changed to produce what we could sell.

In addition to shoring up their own business operations, Zippy's was a driving force for an entrepreneurial effort by the business and travel industries called Movers and Shakas. They received a lot of support from the Hawai'i Executive Collaborative and other local businesses. From their social media platforms, Movers and Shakas "aims to attract socially responsible remote workers to Hawai'i and actively contribute to the community." Their goal is to recruit and nurture "talented professionals to diversify our Hawai'i economy and re-build resilience into our community."

Kirk Caldwell Regarding your Movers and Shakas initiative, how did you get that idea? Were you looking at places like the Caribbean, Aruba, those kinds of places? I would read in the *Economist* about places with these types of ideas that seemed brilliant. In the United States, we've got these restrictions and the Constitution, I thought, *Could we even do the kind of things these other places are doing?* But you grabbed the idea and went with it. How? And why? And what did you believe? And it's not even benefitting your restaurants, really. This is for the community.

Jason Higa There was a number of us from the local business community involved. Denise Yamaguchi was one of the first people I spoke with and then we got on the phone with Duane Kurisu and Colbert Matsumoto and that led to a whole bunch of other people throwing their hats in the ring and saying, "You know, this has potential." Eventually, an advisory board was created that included Ben Ancheta (Inkinen Executive Search), Nā'ālehu Anthony (Hawai'i COVID Collaborative), Lynelle Marble (Hawai'i Executive Collaborative), Rich Matsui (kWh Analytics), Rob Nobriga (Island Holdings, Inc.), Lori Teranishi (iQ 360), Kevin Yim (Zippy's), and Denise Yamaguchi (Hawai'i Agriculture Foundation and Hawai'i Food & Wine Festival).

We were concerned about our hospitality industry, including our hotels and the car rental companies, and all of their employees. So, for all of us, we just wanted to see if we could do something to support the potential for remote work in Hawai'i, especially since Hawai'i was doing so well with the COVID counts at the time compared to other places. We met weekly and eventually came up with Movers and Shakas.

As far as funding, the Department of Business, Economic Development and Tourism provided an early contribution, as they were looking at the potential for remote work in Hawai'i. Each of the advisory board member organizations contributed as well as the Omidyar Ohana Fund and the Kosasa Foundation. United Airlines and Alaska Airlines offered free flights, as they were both also supporting remote work programs in other cities.

Then the timing just worked out perfectly. As we launched Movers and Shakas in November 2020, Hawai'i had the lowest COVID case numbers and the national media was craving a feel-good story. An AP reporter heard of the initiative and offered to release the details of the program to national media. The reporter was going on maternity leave, so we had to set up the Movers and Shakas website, which would accept the online applications. We were able to work with her, and Movers and Shakas hit the national wire with every major media outlet contacting us to learn more about this story. We received over ninety thousand online applicants for fifty openings in a two-week period. The server literally crashed the first weekend, but we were able to fix the issue fairly quickly.

Kirk Caldwell Where was it run out of? Was it here? Out of Zippy's? I look at you as the catalyst, but who did the application process, going to the airlines, finding hotel discounts, and connecting them with projects to help the local community? Who was the laboring oar? Was it you and Zippy's?

Jason Higa It was the advisory board for Movers and Shakas. Each advisory board member contributed toward the development and launch of the program. Upspring Media developed the website. Lynelle Marble kept us on track with all of the tasks and deadlines. Kevin Yim developed the website content and application form. Richard Matsui and Ben Ancheta recruited a volunteer committee to sort and review the ninety thousand applications. Denise Yamaguchi and Nā'ālehu Anthony developed the programs and activities for the fifty cohorts. Lori Teranishi managed all the media inquiries and Rob Nobriga handled the community outreach. Looking back, we didn't have a grand plan on how this was going to work, but we simply put the pieces together week by week.

Kirk Caldwell People volunteered to help farmers and others with technical assistance and other types of skills important to their businesses. Who did the outreach for this?

Jason Higa A number of dynamics were happening, especially during the initial launch of Movers and Shakas. There was an initial community pushback. "Why are you bringing in visitors to Hawai'i during a pandemic? They're going to take our housing," and all sorts of other concerns about the program. One person even wrote an op-ed questioning the program. This person was Nicole Lim, who today is the director of Movers and Shakas.

Nicole had heard about Movers and Shakas from her friends on the Mainland. She submitted her op-ed, which was published in the *Honolulu Star-Advertiser*. Nicole expressed her mixed emotions when she heard about the program. She was concerned about encouraging visitors to Hawai'i during the pandemic, yet she had spent years as a digital nomad traveling the world and visiting almost every country.

A number of advisory board members contacted Nicole and offered her the position to lead Movers and Shakas. She eventually accepted after she began to understand the intent behind the program. Nicole is an amazing woman who has a remarkable educational and professional career. She attended 'Iolani, then Yale University, and earned her MBA at Wharton. She later had a successful career at eBay before becoming a digital nomad for five years. She visited nearly every country, every continent over this five-year period, so she really knew what remote working was like as she continued to do freelance consulting during that period. Finally, as the pandemic started, Nicole's mom asked her to return home to Hawai'i.

Nicole has spearheaded Movers and Shakas and she was the one who developed the strong relationships with all of the community and nonprofit groups, including the PA'I Foundation, Native Hawaiian Hospitality Association and Native Hawaiian Chamber of Commerce, Hawai'i Agricultural Foundation, Future Farmers of America, Work Now Hawaii; Girl Scouts of Hawai'i, North Shore Economic Vitality Partnership, Suma Farms, Nimbus AI, Pacific International Center for High Technology Research, The Pantry by Feeding Hawaii Together, Kamehameha Schools, the DOE, and the Chamber of Commerce Hawai'i. Nicole also carefully matched the right cohorts with the right skillsets with each of the community and nonprofit groups. Without

Nicole, Movers and Shakas would not have succeeded.

There are some incredible outcomes, and some of the cohorts continue to work with their nonprofits. Dante Moore, one of the cohorts, assisted the Native Hawaiian Hospitality Association to develop a website, Kuhikuhi.com, a Yelp for Native Hawaiian–owned businesses. Dante spent enormous amounts of time and continues to do so because it's a passion project for him. Dante is a black entrepreneur who helps minority companies to launch websites, so Kuhikuhi was just perfect for his skillset.

Kirk Caldwell Is he still here in Hawai'i?

Jason Higa No, Dante returned to the Mainland, but continued development on the Kuhikuhi website even after leaving Hawai'i. Another cohort fellow, who also returned to the Mainland, created remote internships for Hawai'i public high school students with his Mainland cybersecurity employer. We are very hopeful that the cohort fellows will return to Hawai'i in the future and renew their connections with the Hawai'i community.

As things started opening up through the tier system, parents and schools made adjustments accordingly. While public schools clearly fell under state jurisdiction under tiers, there was confusion over how independent schools would operate under the City and County orders, which are approved by the governor. Tim Cottrell, 'Iolani School, worked with the DOE and the Hawaii Association of Independent Schools to clarify their position, what they could do, and what they could not do.

Tim Cottrell It was very confusing. We're fortunate to have an attorney on staff who helped review, research, and guide us with regard to the mandates and requirements. We were very rigorous in terms of working within the rules that everybody had set down and were grateful for the exceptions for schools because we were designated as an essential workforce. This allowed us to consider ways to safely modify school activities that would take place in a normal school year. However, we were pretty careful internally about what we classified as a "school activity," as well as taking into account the community conditions at the time of the event.

While we could not, for example, have social activities like the prom, after the forced shutdown in March 2020, we were determined to hold a graduation ceremony as close to normal as possible. We created a beautiful drive-in graduation ceremony on our baseball field that allowed parents to attend with students in their cars, and each student got to walk across the stage to receive their diploma. We developed a rigorous safety plan and submitted the plan to the City and the Honolulu Police Department for approval.

And that's the approach we took with all of our events for the 2020–21 school year. We would write out the safety plan and get approval before moving forward. The process worked and our safety protocols proved effective, because, again, we had things like a modified version of our fair on campus and were able to maintain zero cases of on-campus transmission throughout the entirety of the year.

We also, early on, went through the process of becoming a CLIA-certified testing lab on campus. This allowed us to order tests in bulk, which gave us the ability to test students, faculty, etc., whenever needed. This enabled us to move forward in hosting select school activities in a safe way.

Once vaccinations became available, paired with our ability to rapid test, we very quickly reinstated many school traditions and events. Our seniors were able to have a prom, a senior camp, and a modified ʻIolani Fair we called Raider Fest. It also allowed us to move forward with our graduation ceremony for the class of 2021.

Kirk Caldwell Do you think going through all of this has made the student body at ʻIolani more resilient and connected?

Tim Cottrell I think the experience of everybody having to go through this together and all those trials and travails and everything really made our community stronger. During this time, our faculty and staff voted us as one of the best places to work, and we are proud to have won the

PBN Award as the #1 Best Place to Work in the Large Business category.

Kirk Caldwell What about these major events in your students' young lives? Prom, graduation, sports. How did the students deal with all these things? Did you get pushback from students and parents as you worked through these things? Or did they understand?

Tim Cottrell They understand, and we framed it to not set that expectation. When we lost the quarter of a year, that was in such a period of crisis. Nobody was going to work, everybody was just locked down, so there wasn't really any question of *Why can't we do these things?* The first thing we did was have that drive-in graduation, which people loved. That was a lovely event and our families were very grateful that we made that happen for them.

The following year we were very clear that our goal was to come back on campus and re-establish academic normalcy as much as we could for our students, but we were not trying to be more ambitious than that. You should expect for your child to be able to come to school and do well academically, but we had to wait and see what else could be possible. When the vaccines became available, we were happy to see that our faculty, staff, and students were eager to get the shot. To encourage vaccinations, we hosted a total of seventeen on-campus vaccination clinics in partnership with Safeway. We very quickly reached a 99 percent vaccination rate among our faculty and staff, and a 96 percent vaccination rate among our upper school students, which made it possible for us to consider adding more events back to our schedule. When the vaccine was approved for younger students, we also very quickly achieved a high vaccination rate in our lower school community.

We communicated with our senior class that they were our priority. We told them, "We're going to try to do everything we can to give you the traditional events you would have had." For example, senior camp was delayed, but we were able to hold it in April. So we did a lot of those things. We tried to also work with our peer schools, some of the other private schools, to do what we could in athletics. We offered testing so that our basketball teams could begin to play, and we helped coordinate pickup scrimmages between schools. We were able to test all of the athletes the day of the event to make it possible.

Kirk Caldwell You have your own testing?

Tim Cottrell Yes. We got certified as a CLIA testing lab and I think this was maybe around the turn of the year. We started by ordering about twenty thousand rapid antigen tests. Our ability to test played a significant role in moving forward. Even though we had very high vaccination rates here, we've continued pool testing 25 percent of the school community every week.

Kirk Caldwell At one point I was pushing for pool testing on flights coming in. Just test and see what it shows.

Tim Cottrell That's a good idea. We are also getting a modification to our CLIA certification so that we can use a new test, it's the Abbott ID Now, which is quite a bit more sensitive than the antigen test. With the antigen test, you've got to have COVID for the antigen test to show a positive result. However, with the ID Now test, it is much more sensitive, so you can be just getting it and the ID Now test will show it. Having the ability to conduct both kinds of tests expands our ability to detect asymptomatic cases as well as assist with contact tracing and mitigate the chances of transmission. For example, we can cover a scenario where the difference would be, you're in sixth grade, you test COVID positive, but we really couldn't test the kids with our antigen test because it might take a number of days for them to have enough viral load to be detected, but now we're going to have this ID Now test, where we can test them all immediately. It's very similar to a PCR test. So, we do a lot of testing.

Kirk Caldwell Who had the hardest time? The students, the parents, or the teachers?

Tim Cottrell The teachers. And we totally empathize with that. You're stressed about your own safety, your family's safety, and everything in between. You're coming into something where there's a genuine risk. Then we're putting you in a classroom where you've got a face mask and a face shield on, all your students have a face mask and a face shield on, and you have to communicate with them. So we got microphones. Teachers wore a wireless mic with an amplifier under their face shield so that students could hear them. Then we're saying every classroom has to be accessible to people who are learning temporarily online. So you've got to stream your classroom and be conscious of students who might be online at the same time. It was like running a small television show. I mean, it was super stressful. We did it well, but it was really a lot of work.

To help with that stress, we introduced extra days off throughout the year. We didn't have very many consecutive five-day weeks. If we had a five-day week, we'd drop a Monday or a Friday. This helped tremendously. I think it helped morale, it helped energy, it helped people stay engaged, and it was so popular we continued with four extra days off this year. Everybody recognized the quality of life really goes up when you have just a few more of those days just to manage your life, go to the bank, all those kinds of things for our employees.

Kirk Caldwell Teaching is a lot about communication. Not just your voice, but facial expressions. You can tell if a student is learning or not, and if their faces are covered up the teacher is probably spending even more energy making sure they are connecting with the student and the student is absorbing what is being taught to them.

Tim Cottrell It was draining. And I would watch our teachers in the lower school, and they've got three or four kids online, so they have even more of an impetus to interact with the kids than the upper school teachers. So, they're talking to the kids that are online, they're talking to everybody in class, it was like watching a production of *Sesame Street* or something. Often they would have multiple cameras so they didn't miss any angles. And then of course the work—the homework had to be managed both in-person and online.

As O'ahu managed COVID through the tier system, one of the key medical advisors, Dr. Jonathan Dworkin, who had relocated with his family to the Big Island, immediately got involved with helping Hawai'i Island through Mayor Harry Kim's team. They struggled with some of the same issues, but also faced problems unique to the local communities on that island. He continued to serve on the O'ahu advisory panel and reported to the group weekly.

Jonathan Dworkin (Queen's Health System) I got invited to a couple of Harry Kim's COVID response meetings. It was funny to contrast those with the O'ahu meetings. Harry's a little more eccentric, and he would walk in incensed over Yukio [the outbreak at the Yukio Okutsu State Veterans Home]. He was pissed off. I could tell he was going to have someone's head on a platter for that. But the dynamic here was a little bit different because the ICU resource was far more limited. At the time that I was involved, the two big clusters, there was a nursing home, Yukio—and I think there was one other nursing home at that time when they had a couple of cases identified—and then there was also one in public housing and it was very similar to the Pacific Islander community public housing on the Kona side.

David Derauf and I basically said the same thing when we were speaking with you guys: "You need to get in there. You need to test everybody, separate sick from not sick. You need to try to get a handle on it." They were using Premier to do a lot of their testing and they set up these mobile clinics and they brought in representatives of the Pacific Islander community. Most of those fires ended up being put out. I was worried there was going to be a big wave of cases that was going to hit the hospital hard, but in the end, it was more like a splash than a wave. Most of the nursing home patients went to Hilo Medical Center, not Waimea where I was, or they passed away at the nursing home. But they did eventually get those under control. And they had this benefactor, a Silicon Valley entrepreneur, who was paying for a lot of the testing, so the effort on the Big Island was shaped a little bit differently than O'ahu. It was basically Harry; the Hawaii District Health Office; the tech capital, Premier; and then advice from me as needed. And they didn't need that much because they already had a game plan.

Once Safe Travels started, it changed. Then a lot of it was travel. It was people with a false negative pretravel test or they just got infected after their pretravel test. A lot of them were returning residents. We saw that here and we saw that on O'ahu. At that point, the border control issue became much more salient.

Kirk Caldwell If we would have had testing, tracing, isolation facilities earlier, after the first surge and lockdown, perhaps as we opened back up, we wouldn't have had a surge and a second shutdown. The second shutdown resulted in the City and County of Honolulu doing its own testing with the purchase of a lab located at the airport, massive surge testing, paying for its own contact tracers and isolation facilities at three hotels in Waikīkī. What are your thoughts on this?

Jonathan Dworkin I think the lack of public health definitely hampered us in the summertime. At that point we had a little bit more testing, but not the kind of large-scale screening of asymptomatic high-risk people that I would have really liked. That was not common anywhere at that point. We had practically no contact tracing and I've spoken with Jennifer Smith who's the whistleblower over there and got her version of events. The isolation and quarantine were basically being set up through the City and later on Eddie Mersereau, so I think if we had had a proactive DOH, we certainly would have blunted that second wave.

The tier system that you eventually settled on coming out of the second shutdown was clearly the right thing to do. Earlier, we didn't really have that model and we were just trying to decide in those meetings what's sensible to open up and not sensible to open up. But I think it created a lot of confusion and later on when we had the tier system that sort of depoliticized it and it wasn't *Oh Caldwell is not letting me do this.*

Instead, it was *We're in tier 2 or we're in tier 3.* Earlier, we didn't have that kind of a system and when Blangiardi reviewed your tier system in January that's exactly what I said to him. "Listen, you want to be responsible for every single business that's closed? Because that's what's going to happen to you if you don't have some sort of objective system."

So he kept it around at least until March. I think that was important because it gave us time to vaccinate the highest risk people. So that was a success. We came on a little slowly, but I think it was because we were figuring it out and it was hard to do.

Those were the two things. If we had had really good Singapore-style public health, or even just average public health, and contact tracing services in the summer, we would have been in a better situation and if I could have known about the tier system and advised something like that earlier, that's something I wish I would have done.

Kirk Caldwell Early on, there were no working models of a tier system. But we learned from other forward leaning states and cities what works and what doesn't work. And you're right, it depoliticizes it, and it tells the public what's going to happen, either good or bad, ahead of time.

Jonathan Dworkin We appreciated that you acknowledged that there was a difference of opinion there and that's all we can ask for. Nobody voted for me. That's one of the things I always tell my wife. I'm not the mayor of anything. I'm lucky to be in the room while these conversations are happening. There's always going to be, as the pandemic shifted, trade-offs and difficult decisions to make each time something new happened. When we had testing: *Okay, how do we use the testing?* When we began to open up the border: *What's the best border entry screen?* Now we have vaccinations: *What penetrants of vaccination do we want before we further open?* There's plenty of disagreement on this stuff. Even amongst my *hui* this morning, Tim Brown and Gerry Murphy were having a very spirited argument about how much do we need to vaccinate before we allow the virus to spread more. That kind of a thing. This is a hot topic right now. You have cases going up, but hospitalizations aren't really going up, so is that okay? Do we want to knock down cases? Are there particular populations we need to better protect? So, people don't agree on this stuff and they never did. So you've got to be able to weigh that.

While the images of Waikīkī without people or traffic were breathtaking, a once-in-a-lifetime event, it also meant that Hawai'i's number one industry, tourism, was basically shut down. All visitor industry–related businesses were suffering financial losses and mass unemployment. But perhaps the largest financial loss on a per day average was being reported by Hawaiian Airlines. Peter Ingram described his days as CEO, and his efforts to lead the airline through its darkest time.

Georgette Deemer I think the most dramatic statistic that I heard during the whole pandemic was the amount of financial loss that the airlines were taking, far greater than a hotel or a business or a restaurant or whatever. I mean, your losses were phenomenal.

Peter Ingram In the second quarter last year, we were burning through cash at a pace of $3.5 million a day.

Georgette Deemer I'm thinking, *Is Hawaiian going to survive?* But then you talked about borrowing money. Now, who do you borrow from? From the government? Or from some other entity?

Peter Ingram So ultimately, we've raised about $2.2 billion over the course of the pandemic—$388 million of that was from federal government programs through the CARES Act and the Payroll Support Program, and there have been two extensions to that. So that's less than 20 percent of the total.

Georgette Deemer Do you have to pay that back?

Peter Ingram A portion of it is a loan and a portion of it was a grant as long as we fulfilled all the terms. The rest of what we've raised is all loans, so through major financial institutions we raised money through an enhanced equipment trust certificate (EETC). Effectively, a mortgage on aircraft. So that was a few hundred million dollars. We did a $1.2 billion loan—our largest borrowing ever—that was collateralized by our loyalty program. That was a public debt offering, an offer to institutional investors. So most of it was private market raising money, and the market for that got a lot better when people could see the light at the end of the tunnel. Back in April, May, June last year, there wasn't really anyone that wanted to talk to us about lending.

One, we had the federal government, and the other thing we had was a revolving credit facility, which is an outstanding piece of debt that you can call on, and that was a pretty easy decision. Okay, we're going to just draw that down. In our case, that was $225 million of buffer.

But you're right. When you're burning through $3.5 million a day—and we started last year with something like $700 million in the bank and we never really want to go below about $400 million or $500 million. Some of our debt agreements, we couldn't go below $300 million or bad financial things start to happen. It's not too hard to do the math. We can't do this forever, so we have to stop that cash burn by controlling our spending because we weren't doing it by raising revenue.

By the third quarter, that cash burn number started to come down. As we got to the end of the first quarter this year, we're now at a point where cash inflows/cash outflows were about the same. We'll swing more into the positive when we get the international business up and running again.

Kirk Caldwell I can't believe you're smiling when you talk about this.

Peter Ingram Part of the reason I'm smiling is—I'll tell you. I think back to a year ago at this time and it was terrible. We didn't have a prospect for…

Kirk Caldwell A vaccine? They were doing tests, trials. We didn't know when the trials would be completed and when the multiple government approvals would be given to use the vaccines. But you got through it and you're smiling now. But back then, you're looking at your cash flow, you're borrowing money, you're balancing revenue and expenses, and you have no idea how long the pandemic is going to last, you don't know if the vaccine is going to work, you don't know when it's going to be approved, you don't know how it's going to get distributed, none of that is known. And you're making decisions on...

Peter Ingram As a layman, last summer, if you'd have asked me about whether I was counting on vaccines as being the ticket out of this, I'm like, *Vaccines take too long to develop, right?* That was our historic paradigm. And there were coronaviruses for which there's never been a vaccine developed. So I was thinking, I'm one who always bets on the scientists to solve problems, but I was betting it would be more on therapeutics than the vaccine. The vaccine seemed like too much of a long shot to me to make a bet on last year.

Georgette Deemer I think everybody was very relieved because we knew that you had a financial background, so you came into this position with a good head for your financial situation. Since people have been flying again, it seems like the airline customer culture has changed. People are much more violent, angry, or not friendly.

Peter Ingram We've seen some of this and a lot of it centers around the enforcement of the mask policy, which was more rigorously enforced first by airlines and then it became a federal guideline. All the airlines had imposed a mask requirement around the time when the CDC began recommending it, at least by the middle of the year. I think people are more nervous about interacting with other people, and so when you get to public gathering places at a time when no one was gathering publicly, I think that just heightened some tensions, but we haven't had as many egregious examples as some of the other carriers. Partially because our flights for a while weren't as full, but now we're operating a lot of full flights again. I think there's been a general level of incivility and I can't put my finger on exactly what the cause of that is, but we just can't tolerate that in our environment.

As routinely as we take safety in the airline industry, it's only routine because we work every day to make sure it stays that way. So we can't have that sort of behavior and we've been very supportive of the Federal Aviation Administration and others stepping in to support us so we can make sure there are consequences for people who do misbehave in that environment.

Maui County also experienced problems between visitors and residents when the island opened up again to out-of-state travelers.

Mike Victorino (Mayor of Maui County) Our local residents were able to enjoy their beaches and minimal traffic during the lockdowns. Even Hāna wasn't busy because no one was going out there except for the residents and some businesses that provide essential services out there. So Maui County people got used to that. Then the visitors came back with a vengeance. There was a lot of pent-up demand and for some reason Maui was really, really targeted. People wanted to come to Maui. And Maui has a good reputation. What I witnessed was it was too much, too quickly. We weren't prepared for it. Our businesses struggled because they couldn't get enough employees and so service and the quality of experience had dropped somewhat and that's the last thing we want—for our visitors to have a bad experience.

The anti-visitor sentiment has been higher on Maui than in other parts of the state, but I know throughout the state, residents felt like the tourists just took back everything—the beaches and the parks. I think most people felt that way.

For us it was good for the economy because it really helped a lot of our restaurants, hotels, all the ancillary services, the scuba divers, the surfing lessons. It all came back and came back very strong. However, the residents in general are really upset about our inability to control the volume of visitors. The Road to Hāna is under control now, but we had to install new signs out there, forbid parking in many areas, send police out to manage traffic and restrict the number of people going into certain areas, like Wai'ānapanapa.

So we've been trying to balance increased visitor demand with the well-being of our residents. Maui had more visitors than O'ahu during that time. We could combine visitors to Kaua'i and Hawai'i Island together and we'd still be like two or three thousand ahead of them. So it was good and bad. A mixed bag. Good for the economy, but disappointing for the residents because we had been warned that tourism wouldn't recover until late 2022, early 2023. And here by May, June, July of 2021, tourism is at pre-pandemic numbers.

Kirk Caldwell I was reading in the *Star-Advertiser* that out in the Hāna area, local residents, Native Hawaiians in particular, were putting up cones to control traffic and parking to assist visitors but were being sworn at and told to F-off by visitors. They said, "We're up here just trying to control the chaos, but a lot of angry people coming from the continent are being rude to us when it's our home." Did you get pulled into trying to find the balance and get visitors to be more respectful and more *pono*?

Mike Victorino Like I shared with our residents, aloha is something we share with the world and it's important we continue to share it. My response to the visitors: "This is our community, Maui is not a theme park. It's not like Disneyland or Disney World for you to come and enjoy, and then go home. This is our community. If you can't respect our culture and respect our way of life, then don't come. We want you to be respectful to our culture, our lifestyle, and, most importantly, to our resources. Not just destroying everything or trampling over our beaches and trails. Being respectful is very important. We don't need you here creating more havoc for our residents in the middle of a pandemic. This is where we live. We don't have another choice. We live here, so please be respectful of our community." That's the message I tried to put out there.

And so, yes, I got some backlash, you saw in the paper, *Mayor Victorino Says, "Don't Come,"* but they didn't print the rest of the message. Because the lack of respect to our culture and our resources and our community, I didn't want them coming.

Kirk Caldwell Well, I thought you showed courage standing up for your community. I liked it.

Mike Victorino Like everything else, Kirk, you get those who liked it and you get those who thought I was crazy. My own staff said, "No, don't say that." But it was a message that needed to be said. And even now I tell people if you can't respect our culture and our way of life, don't come—we are in the middle of a pandemic. The infection numbers are astronomically high. Our hospital, our medical facility, our medical staff, our healthcare workers can't afford another surge. They're tired. They're worn out. And now there are more cases than ever. At the same time, we have tourists who go out and go up on trails and get hurt, break their leg, get hurt in the ocean, and it just adds to the trauma of what our healthcare system is experiencing. We need to address this by saying maybe there should be a slowdown of visitor arrivals. I don't know, something must be done. We're at wits end at this point. Capacity is being exceeded in many of our hospitals throughout the state of Hawai'i.

Kirk Caldwell You've used the term "knuckleheads" in describing these disrespectful people and the press has picked it up and quoted you on it quite a bit. It's an old-fashioned term, but you brought it back.

Mike Victorino Yes, a lot of people out there are knuckleheads, in many respects, in parts of our community. They don't seem to care about others.

Kirk Caldwell And one thing I wanted to circle back to—you're the mayor of three islands, inhabited islands, the only mayor with that responsibility, and each island is very different from the other. And for me on O'ahu, I just have to worry about one island, and yeah there's different communities on it, but you have some very distinct communities. How did you handle that? How did you find the balance to address the unique needs of each of those islands?

Mike Victorino Knowing your community is very important. I think every mayor works so hard to understand their communities. I have three inhabited islands. I even consider Hāna almost a complete separate island because of the distance, isolation, and where it's located. Understanding their desires and needs, getting in there during the first outbreak was really important. First, showing that I cared enough when we went in and had entire towns sanitized, like Molokaʻi and Hāna, and other areas in Wailuku and Kahului. We took every appropriate action we knew at that time to slow the virus down to prevent people from getting sick. And I don't think anybody can say I didn't really try to protect my community every time the call was made.

John De Fries became the executive director of the Hawaiʻi Tourism Authority (HTA) in the fall of 2020, starting on the same day that Dr. Libby Char started as the new director of health. Both assumed critical positions at the height of the pandemic.

Kirk Caldwell John, I don't know you well on a personal level. But as mayor, when we'd be on these Zoom calls and listening to you even now, you come across as a very calm and kind person. You don't react quickly or strongly to opposing views and you're in a very controversial business right now. There is a strong anti-tourism element saying there are too many tourists. You have the visitor industry pressuring you to bring more visitors here. You have a business community who realizes it's so important to have those visitors or they're not going to survive, such as our restaurant industry, which in large part is dependent on the visitors returning in large numbers. On top of that, the legislature has significantly cut your funding. And yet, you don't let it get to you. I have not heard you say, "I took this job at the wrong time." How do you manage that?

John De Fries If I was twenty-five or thirty years younger, and less experienced, I'd be out of my mind right now. Because when we're younger, we don't make the distinctions well between what it is we can control and what we can't control. So therefore, we go about trying to control it all and we burn ourselves out as we hemorrhage our mana, creativity, and patience.

A high school friend, a classmate, said to me, "John, right about now people in our class are retiring and you decided to go jump into this leadership role at HTA." This classmate was trying to understand my mindset, so I responded by saying, "You know, I don't run as fast and I don't jump as high, because I don't need to." Once you make an assessment and you understand the forces at work, you can identify the pathways that enable you to move forward.

There were a number of people this past week who wanted me to publicly challenge Governor Ige's statement about visitors not traveling to Hawaiʻi at this time. My response was, "Look, once the chief executive of the state makes the decision, whether I agree with it or not is irrelevant. What will exasperate the situation is if I get into a public debate with the governor and it becomes a storyline picked up by global media that then depicts this divisiveness between the visitor industry and state government. And where is that going to get us?"

Our governor, you as mayor of Honolulu, and your colleague mayors on our Neighbor Islands have to make tough decisions each and every day in balancing the health and safety of our communities with the restart and stabilization of our economic recovery. And, frankly, I was honored to have HTA support all of you through these tough times.

You know, I don't have to go very far, I don't even have to go outside my family, to hear concerns and comments about tourism. So in real time, all I have to do is talk to my family members or neighbors or open the daily paper or pick up my mobile device to get a feel for the community landscape and resident sentiments. But, as Native Hawaiians or as kamaʻāina, we're not going anywhere. It's not like, oh, I'm fed up so I'm going to leave. That's not even part of our makeup. So we've got to be able to make it work by finding a balance between the well-being of our communities, the health and protection of our natural resources, and the economic vitality that is infused by the visitor industry.

In tourism, the journey of the visitor is one where he or she is moving through multiple levels of regulatory jurisdiction. From arriving at a state airport being operated under state and federal auspices, then getting on a state highway, turning down a county road, checking into a hotel on private property, and the next day visiting a county beach or a state park. So the perception that managing tourism comes under a single institution is flawed. If there is a single institution it's called the State of Hawaiʻi coupled with each of the four counties, because it's a matter of us being able to convene each of the jurisdictions, to coordinate and collaborate and come up with solutions. This, I see, as being central to HTA's function.

People say, "Well, HTA doesn't have much authority." And I say, "Let's assume I have no authority." It doesn't prevent me from convening and collaborating with those who do have the authority and help them think this through. It doesn't need to be my solution. So in that respect, I'm really kind of comfortable with working that way and moving fluidly between different agencies and learning about their capabilities and limitations as a means of arriving at a collaborative set of solutions. In this area, we still have a ways to go. *

CHAPTER 6

Hope in a Vaccine

At the end of 2020, the Pfizer and Moderna COVID vaccines were cleared to be administered in the United States. This created great hope that the vaccine was going to be the best tool to help us successfully manage the virus, if not eradicate it. The Johnson & Johnson vaccine became available a few months later in early 2021. The vaccine triggered changes around the world in many ways. It allowed government to rethink the need for restrictions, doctors and healthcare workers to consider the effectiveness of the vaccine over time, and played heavily in the opening of schools, hospitals, businesses, public gatherings, and workplaces based on vaccination status.

There were and continue to be misperceptions, both positive and negative, on what the vaccine can actually do. Society became deeply divided between those who were vaccinated, those who were hesitant, and those who refused to get vaccinated for personal and/or political reasons. As a result, the virus continued to stay alive, spread, and mutate throughout the world. What started as placing all of our hopes on the vaccine has evolved into resignation that we may be wrestling with COVID for an indeterminate amount of time, and that boosters and new vaccines will need to be developed to fight each new variant that emerges.

Leading the state on vaccination policy is Dr. Libby Char, director of health, starting with addressing the misinformation on why someone would opt not to get vaccinated.

Libby Char (Hawaiʻi DOH) Some people said this is just like the flu, especially for young people, it's just like the flu. They ignored the long-term devastation that can come from COVID and the fact that people would die from infections with this virus. The long-term sequelae affects you neurologically. We know that it can affect your heart and lungs, we know that there can be lingering effects, and for people to say if you get sick it's like the flu, it's like a cold—why would you condemn somebody to that knowing that we can mitigate the amount of disease in the community and morbidity in the cases? We can do things to help mitigate that.

And again, you have to balance the public health side with the economic side, and there are other factors that have to be weighed, but I think it's flawed thinking that *Oh, I don't think it's that bad—we don't need to be concerned about people getting infected.*

The whole point of the vaccination was even if you do get it, it won't be as severe. Your chances of dying are significantly less, your chances of getting severe illness and ending up in the hospital in the ICU on a ventilator are significantly lower, but it's not zero.

And now that we're seeing these variants come in, that's really starting to rework that thinking because the number of breakthrough cases, the amount of illness that we're seeing in relation to these variants, it's really putting us on notice. One of the things I'm grateful to the governor for is that he made some difficult and unpopular decisions. They weren't the easy decisions, but they were the right decisions and he kept some of the mitigation measures in place while others were clamoring to remove all the restrictions even when it wasn't indicated. We were catching a lot of flak about CDC and indoor masking after they removed the guidance to wear masks indoors for those who had gotten vaccinated, but it didn't make sense to us and the governor kept it in place. Some people didn't understand and became upset about that. We were trying to get the message out, but sometimes I think people don't want to understand, they don't want to hear it. They are going to hear what they want to hear.

We started seeing more and more breakthrough cases. And if you look at Israel, they have a similar vaccination rate to the state of Hawai'i and they're having significant breakthrough cases from the Delta variant. And they're finding that their most vulnerable are the older citizens and that's why they're starting to talk about doing a booster shot for the older population. That's why we are hanging on to "wear your masks indoors." That will probably be the last thing to go. We know it's effective. And even if people have been vaccinated, there's still a risk, indoors, and that risk is growing as we see these variants coming in. We're seeing more and more breakthroughs: people who are fully vaccinated get exposed and get infected.

People are calling it vaccine failure. It's not a failure of the vaccine. The vaccine is doing exactly what it was designed to do—prevent severe illness and death. It's not one hundred percent. We know that people will get sick. And that's one of the things right now with some of the counties wanting to have mega gatherings. It should be safer if everybody's vaccinated, but statistically if you have enough people at a gathering, there will be cases that result from that gathering.

What if your event that created that environment caused people to become sick? What are you going to do about it? What are you going to do for that person? That's another current frustration. That event organizer doesn't take responsibility for it. It becomes a DOH responsibility.

Someone else has to take care of isolation/quarantine. Someone else has to take care of contact tracing. Someone else has to take care of feeding people in quarantine and isolation, housing them, and making sure they have wraparound services. Really?

Trying to convey that this is not a good idea, it puts you at odds with somebody. They see you as opposition. And it's like, you don't get it, do you? We're all part of this community. This is my city too. I live here. I'm part of this community. I'm not your enemy, I just want our community to be healthy and safe.

The counties, especially City and County of Honolulu, really stepped up, wanted to help, intended to help, and did help. And that was from the very beginning. Remember in the federal surge testing? Honolulu Fire Department totally stepped up and helped pull that off. That was a mammoth lift. Six days to go from having the discussion to actually having people drive up and get tested. That was huge because it showed that it could be done. At the time, the State wasn't able to do it, and the County stepped up and said we're doing it. And they all looked at you like you were nuts because it was six days—something that should take two months to plan. And the fire department with the help of the Honolulu Police Department and some others pulled it off. That was huge and it showed that we could do something. It helped pave the way for the rollout of vaccinations.

Kirk Caldwell I thought that as well. So you believed that too?

Libby Char Yes, because we knew that we had a model now and that we could do something on this scale. Even if it didn't end up looking exactly like that, we knew that we could pull something off and that it should involve the City and those who had a bigger reach and a bigger lift, and that we should partner with them. That was really important. We referenced that when we were crafting the whole vaccination program to form these bonds, these partnerships with the City and County. The State doesn't have a ton of people for the operational side of things, the City and County does. They had not only incident management, but big IMTs (incident management teams), so the State and City worked collaboratively. We knew we had to partner and work together if we were going to get this done. And that's what happened. Especially on this island.

When you talk about the economy, again, it's like we're at odds; we're the bad guy making too many rules. How much economic loss will there be if you get an infection in your kitchen staff and now you don't have anybody to show up for work? You have to close your whole restaurant down for at least two weeks. How much of an economic toll will that result in? We have a responsibility to try and keep the employees safe and healthy as well. Let's use all the mitigation measures we can so people are healthy to go to work and can also be in a safe environment.

We know more and more of the science surrounding COVID. We see the clusters in certain trades or categories, or circumstances. We have had several clusters involving employees in restaurants. It can be a hot, crowded environment; people are close together and tend to not be wearing masks a lot of the time. It would have been helpful for all of the restaurants to encourage and incentivize their members to get vaccinated.

Kirk Caldwell And another one is *Why do you make us wear masks?*

Libby Char There was a degree of shortcomings being someone else's fault. There's some sort of fault involved. Many said they were being punished by having to wear masks. They talked about fault and how the DOH wouldn't let them do something, or that the DOH was making them do something, and it's such a false narrative. It's not me that's causing these problems. It's a virus called SARS-CoV-2, but people sometimes only see an adversarial situation. Let's identify the DOH as the bad guy, or public health or the medical community as the bad guy. And that's really frustrating.

If your industry is so concerned about this, why don't you do more about it? I was reading about a company called Wahine Builders. I think they required their employees to be vaccinated. It cost them, I think, two employees who quit. But they required it and I applaud them for taking action to keep the rest of their employees safe. They know that when they show up for work, every one of their coworkers is vaccinated. When they're riding to the worksite, they know they are all vaccinated, which means a safer environment and less chance of someone getting infected. When they're having lunch, they're all safer. They're still wearing masks, they're still distanced, but they can feel safer knowing that their employer cares enough to make sure they have a safe work environment.

Incentivize the heck out of your employees, require it where you can. Props to Wahine Builders for doing that. Why don't other companies do it? We made the vaccine available, we made these guys priority populations for some of the essential workers, and when we're doing case investigations on outbreaks and clusters, we're asking the crew with the infected coworkers and we find out that only 40 percent of them are vaccinated. We made them a priority group and we made the vaccine available for them as best we could at no cost to them.

We continue to hear this narrative of "somebody else won't let us do something" or "somebody else is making us do something." We're all in the same community, guys. Stop complaining about how the public health folks are making life difficult for you. Be positive instead. Do something about it! Go get your team vaccinated. Encourage it. Incentivize them if they get vaccinated. I don't know, whatever it takes. Give them a day off, two days off. But the businesses really have that within their purview, their control. They could incentivize.

Understand, there's always going to be a population that will not, but there's a lot of study and research out there that shows that if you incentivize, at a certain point, people will buy in. If I told you you could have a week of paid vacation to get vaccinated, I think people would be interested in that. It's going to cost, but the point is you could figure out what it would take to get your people vaccinated.

Jonathan Dworkin (Queen's Health System) The vaccine efficacy is still really good for severe disease, but it's not perfect. We're seeing some vaccinated people get sick; we had our first death not long ago. The efficacy for symptomatic disease might be a little bit lower than it was a few months ago. We're seeing clusters now of vaccinated people that get mildly ill, which is a little bit new. In countries with good vaccine programs, like the UK, they are having a big surge in infection, so you've got to wonder are some of these vaccinated people transmitting asymptomatically and what does that do to the pandemic over time? So I think it has shifted again a little bit. We're probably going to need a booster, and if we don't synchronize that with getting vaccines to the developing world, then we're going to be in a situation where we're having to boost all the time because we're importing from god knows where some new mutant strain.

What I really hope for is that federal leadership is focusing on 1) when do we boost and working all the details on when we roll that out, and 2) how do we synchronize that with the global vaccination effort? Because what you saw in early 2021 was tremendous success of the vaccination program. We really knocked it out well.

But it's coming back in, now with variants from places that were neglected. I think that's going to be the main thing for the next year or so. And until that happens, we can't just stop doing public health. We still need to have, ideally, some system of border control for the state of Hawai'i, some ability to test, trace, isolate.

The counter argument is I think as long as the hospital is not full, we'll just let it rip and we'll get to herd immunity faster. But the downside consequence of that is what you just articulated, which is that we could end up dealing with a much worse epidemic later because we've allowed it to spread and mutate in a partly vaccinated population. So I think I'm with Tim Brown and with the majority on this particular one. I'd like to see us knock it down until we can get the vaccine to the world.

Kirk Caldwell Another important component is mask wearing. I admire the governor's holding the line on this protocol. CDC says you don't need to if you're vaccinated. How do you know who's vaccinated and how hard is it to wear a mask? You get these restaurant guys who say it's hard for their workers to wear a mask. Well, workers in some parts of the world were wearing masks way before COVID-19.

WHY DO CERTAIN PEOPLE REFUSE TO GET THE VACCINE?

David Derauf (Kōkua Kalihi Valley) Well, there's politics, but I think there's a lot of other things involved. My own take, talking to friends in the Pacific Islander community, is that there's just a long history of distrust. We have not bridged that community well still. They feel like, You haven't been here for me, ever. Why am I going to trust you now? You say you're here for me. You've never been here for me before. I think there's a lot of that. There's that in Kalihi still too. They say, "I don't know you. I don't like what you're selling. You've never been there for me before."

What works for me with the vaccine—and I mostly deal with the vaccine hesitant, not the resistant—it is exactly what I think you would do, Mayor. You would sit down with the person and hear them out. What's going on? How are you, first of all? Right? The basics! How are you doing? What's going on in your life? Because this virus might not be as big compared to "My son is in court next week—I'm worried about it, Doc." Okay, I'm going to hear you out about that first. Maybe then we'll come around to the vaccine. *Hey, has anyone talked to you about this vaccine?* "Well, yeah, I heard at church that it's not such a good idea." Okay, what did they say? What do you think about that? What would it take to change your mind? You're not ready today. You want to come back next week, we'll talk about it again? That's what it's taking. It's really one by one. Slow by slow. It's happening. Yesterday, we had a big group come in to get the vaccine.

I hate what's happening now. Because I see people vilifying them: these are bad people who aren't getting vaccinated. No, they're not bad people. Those are our neighbors, those are our friends, those are our community members. If we lose our trust in one another and our care for one another, we're sunk. We're sunk with this thing. We've got to build bridges and we have to pull together. As hard as that is.

One thing I've learned in this last year, if we lose that trust, we got nothing. The minute you start fighting, the minute you start blaming someone, you start to lose that trust. That and acknowledge what we might not know and where we make mistakes. You know, Mayor, you owned up to mistakes. You did. And that wasn't an easy thing to do. I saw you do that. "I made a mistake. If I could go back, I wouldn't do it that same way." We need a lot more of that humility right now. If there's anything I've learned, it's just be humble about what we know and don't know. We're going to make mistakes. It's an emergency. None of us have been through this before. This is the first time we're getting tested like this. Can we learn something from that?

For me, learning is all about just being. Realizing that number one, science is not about having the answers. That's a big part of it for me. Science is about asking the right set of questions. Are we asking the right set of questions yet? Don't tell me you got the answers. You don't. Ten years from now someone will say that was all nonsense. We didn't know what we were doing. You know that's going to be the case. We'll look back ten years and if we're alive, we'll say, "How could we have been thinking that?" What we don't know is a lot. We should acknowledge that.

That's also in medicine. You don't go into the room saying, for example, "I know this vaccine is right for you. Why are you not getting vaccinated? How ignorant and stupid of you." That's not going to be very helpful. "Uh, I'll see you later. I'm not coming into your vaccine clinic."

Our vaccine clinics, I wish you could have seen them. They were welcoming, sitting people down, getting them water, nice music—it was lovely. Other people from the National Guard and from the fire department who took part in it were like, "Hey, more of them should be like this. People are having fun here."

Duane Kurisu spoke about the challenges of getting the low-income and the homeless communities vaccinated.

Georgette Deemer I was thinking how, on the west side, they have the lowest rate of vaccinations, and somebody said it's because they don't trust government, they don't believe government has their best interest in mind, so if they're pushing vaccination it must mean that "I don't want it." Do you sense that at all within Kahauiki Village?

Duane Kurisu (Hawai'i Executive Collaborative) When I talked to Connie Mitchell, CEO of the Institute for Human Services, for her opinion on this matter, she agreed that there is some of that, but that we also need to take into consideration how much of a role culture plays in their decision too. For example, in getting the Marshallese, the Micronesians, who were recent immigrants to understand our health-care practices is a challenge. Culturally, some of them still think that getting the vaccine meant that they are sick.

But I'm glad you said what you said about people not trusting government because that's what I feel about this whole thing. I was supposed to be on TV for a press conference for Hawai'i vaccinations to give away Giants tickets as one of the incentives. In retrospect, I was glad that I had a conflict in schedule and couldn't attend the press conference. If I did, I would have said, "I'm giving the tickets only because I was asked to. I don't know why we have to give people something as an incentive for them to think about helping protect their own family, friends, and neighbors. What happened to Hawai'i? We're supposed to be thinking about each other. That's what made us special. What happened to us?"

This further emphasizes the need for us to focus on building community. For us older guys, we cannot forget what we had—communities where people cared for each other, communities that were built upon trust, dignity, and pride. With the Hawai'i Executive Collaborative (HEC), we have embarked on starting to fulfill that vision by focusing on Ka'ū as the foundation for building resilient communities in rural areas throughout Hawai'i. We started with the district of Ka'ū because it has some of the lowest socioeconomic metrics in the state, and it also has some of the most committed and action-driven community leaders. We named the project the Ka'ū Dream.

Starting with Ka'ū High School as the hub, the HEC raised funds to help deepen and broaden Ka'ū High School's reach inside and outside the district through new hires for workforce development, entrepreneurship, summer school and certification programs with Hawai'i Community College, which will allow students and adults to earn their AA degree from Ka'ū High School. We are helping to bring in KTA Superstores to Ka'ū to allow its residents to purchase basic needs at reasonable prices, building art like we see in Kaka'ako, and commitments for music from professional musicians on the island. There are other schools in Hawai'i that allow earned college credits in high school, but the difference in Ka'ū is that it is all community based. In Ka'ū Dream, it's about community building community.

So to answer your question about the leeward side, I think it starts with community. Getting the community engaged and then believing again in their future, in the future of institutions, and, eventually, government building public trust and allowing all of us to believe in government again.

Kirk Caldwell Perhaps the success rate of the vaccination program would have been better if it was community driven instead of top-down from government. If it's coming holistically from the community, like your Ka'ū effort, then it's in all our interests to get vaccinated. It's your neighbor suggesting you get vaccinated because they're concerned about you and themselves too.

Duane Kurisu I'm not an expert on this subject matter, but perhaps if the initiative was built organically, maybe the vaccination rate could have been higher. I don't know. But to overcome the rapid spread of COVID-19, time was not our friend. In times of crisis, immediate action at transformational speed and not organic growth could be top of mind. Another cloud that I think we might consider whenever there are such strong opinions that fracture our society, perhaps we might want to consider who could gain by being smarter about disinformation whether they be forces, inside and outside the US, that purposefully encourages divisiveness.

Kirk Caldwell David Derauf talks about vaccine mandates creating a division in the community. And he sees it within families where marriages are at a breaking point because one spouse won't get vaccinated. He believes it is the worst thing that could happen right now. You got to approach it in a different way where you're not causing division.

VACCINATIONS AND EDUCATION

Christina Kishimoto's challenge was to get thirteen thousand teachers and forty-three thousand employees within the DOE vaccinated, and then to get the message out to the community.

Christina Kishimoto (Hawai'i DOE) We created a team that was going to actually be at vaccine sites. So they were alongside the healthcare workers and HI-EMA, and the various police departments. I came out for several of these and our staff was there too because we wanted to create confidence in our employees. We're there when you get there. You're going to see a face that's familiar. And so, what was great is that all of our partners said it's a good idea, so why don't we create a DOE table? So at the DOE table, we had our communications team, all familiar faces. We had Phyllis Unebasami, who's our deputy superintendent, so people recognized some of these people either from the media or articles or things that we send out internally.

People got the word out very quickly. I went out and got my vaccine.

Online, people said, "Hey, Supe's (superintendent) getting it too," and it just created this phone call, a lot of people calling other people saying, "Yeah, you should get it. You should get it."

And we got a lot of people vaccinated. Twenty-two thousand employees out of over forty thousand vaccinated at our tables. Which meant that we knew that half of our employees were vaccinated. We knew that some went to their own doctors or other sites. We're not privy to that information. Even to this day, we don't know—we're not supposed to collect health information. DOH was the primary partner, along with every other health provider.

Kirk Caldwell And getting kids vaccinated. Was it the Hawai'i Pacific Health vaccination bus that would go to schools and immunize those twelve and older?

Christina Kishimoto We have tons of vaccine sites for the kids. The entire May and June (2021), we did every island. When CDC announced that twelve and over could get it, we had a vaccine site open. We were that quick, and then we had to shut it down because we were too quick. We needed it in writing. So we delayed that one by twenty-four hours, and for two months we've been vaccinating kids. And again, because this is a partnership with each of the healthcare providers and they are the only ones that can own that information, we can't keep sign ins, we can't keep anything like that. We don't have names or numbers or anything right now, but we've done tons of vaccinations.

Kirk Caldwell Can they come by themselves or do they have to come with a parent?

Christina Kishimoto We had a process if they were going to come without a parent. They had to have the appropriate forms signed and filed, but we asked them to come with parents because we were trying to vaccinate the whole family. So we said not only can a child come, but you can also bring all your aunties and everyone with that child's registration. We did a ton of people, which is great. I'm proud of this work. The lives that were saved. I keep telling my team, "You should be really proud that you served the community. You had your hands full this entire time in service." We had fifty-four vaccination sites on O'ahu and four more coming.

David Lassner (University of Hawai'i) I believe we were the first entity in the state to announce a vaccination requirement. This was at the recommendation of our Health and Wellbeing Working Group. We had to think through how to implement a mandate like this. We had implemented a pretty app that supported a daily health check for students and employees who were coming to campus. That software was updated to let everyone upload their vaccination cards. It shows clearance on a single screen if you've verified you are symptom-free and if you've been vaccinated or had a negative test within the last seven days. And it will give you a green light to come on campus or enter a building if you've done that.

Kirk Caldwell So if you're not vaccinated but you are getting tested every seven days, then you're okay?

David Lassner For this fall only. We naively thought at least one of the vaccines would be fully approved over the summer, but we backed off when it turned out the vaccines were under emergency use authorization only as we were preparing for the semester. So we provided the testing option as an alternative and integrated test results into our app as well.

Kirk Caldwell Is it a test that the student has to pay for?

David Lassner We're paying for testing with federal relief funds and offer tests on campus. We know that our requirements have been challenging to our community but our numbers show our efforts are working. Our employees are close to 95 percent vaccinated, and our students will be over 90 percent very shortly, and I think with the Pfizer test approved today, we'll get students pretty close to 95 percent. So we'll be one of the safest places in the state.

We have a lot of nervous people, especially faculty, concerned about whether it is safe to be here. I haven't been getting complaints today, but probably some people are. We think it will settle in. It's like a lot of these things—it's rocky the first day.

Kirk Caldwell To get the test, for example, at UH Mānoa, do they go to one place?

David Lassner We're conducting our vaccination program out of our student health center. That's another area where we invested federal relief dollars to increase capacity. Many students and employees also took advantage of private vaccination options.

Kirk Caldwell Tim, on the vaccine, you said faculty was over 99 percent vaccinated and the upper school was about 96 percent.

Tim Cottrell ('Iolani School) Because the lower school can't get vaccinated, yet. So upper school, seventh to twelfth, I think we're at 96.5 percent.

Kirk Caldwell Amazing. How are you approaching those who are resisting getting vaccinated? For example, Dr. David Derauf of Kōkua Kalihi Valley believes that pushing mandates is creating a division in our community and a shaming of some sort is taking place. He advises that while we're better than most places because of 'ohana, we still can split our community apart if we don't approach this issue with greater sensitivity. Do you find that with students? The shaming or fear of being ostracized?

Tim Cottrell So maybe two things on that point. We made it very easy, comparatively, to get an exemption. Normally, it's quite difficult if you look at whatever it is these days. The State requires twenty-four or twenty-five vaccinations for different purposes. It's not easy to get an exemption these days. If you want the religious exemption, you must have never gotten a vaccine. If you've gotten one, you're excluded from claiming that exemption. So if for whatever religious reasons you don't want your child to get the HPV vaccine that's mandated now by the DOE and they haven't done it but they got their polio vaccine, you're out. So we didn't do that at all. We made it very easy. We don't challenge somebody if they have a religious exemption. And on the medical side, we said you don't need a medical condition. You can just have your pediatrician write a letter stating this family does not want their child to get vaccinated.

But even with that flexibility, we didn't see people resisting the vaccine. In our upper school, only about forty-five out of 1,400 students asked for an exemption. And we were careful not to single kids out. That's why we haven't done anything other places are doing, which is to say if you're not vaccinated you go into a special testing protocol. I don't think that's okay. So we're statistically reaching a level where it's okay for us to have forty-five kids out of 1,400 walking around not vaccinated. When you put them in clusters, you think the virus wants to go from one person to another; well they're surrounded primarily by vaccinated people and they're wearing masks, so there aren't many places for the virus to go. So, statistically, that's the way it should be. And then we're doing all that pool testing, so they're just part of the larger group. Kids who aren't vaccinated are not being singled out or anything like that because again, with teenagers, you don't want to put any kid in a position like that.

BUSINESS AND THE VACCINE

Chris Benjamin (Alexander & Baldwin) The thing that worries me is that this vaccine has allowed us to almost pretend that the pandemic is over. This pandemic is not over. This pandemic may not be over for years. What we have to hope and pray is that the vaccination rate in the United States is high enough that we can keep it at a sustainable level. We're just lucky that the vaccine seems to be effective against the Delta variant. Imagine if the next Theta variant, or whatever's coming next, isn't immune to the vaccine.

Kirk Caldwell We must also make sure that we vaccinate the rest of the world. Richer countries need to do more. Otherwise, the Indias and the Brazils of the world, if their populations are not adequately vaccinated, will cause mutations that may be immune to the developed vaccines. Can you imagine having to go back again? There's no way we could do that. And then you've got all the people in our country who won't get vaccinated.

Paul Yonamine (Central Pacific Bank) I went through an emotional roller coaster through the whole vaccine process. Today, I'm not sure if all those emotions were worth it. We still don't know what's going to happen with COVID long term. And I think that while it is easy to criticize people's choices—a lot easier because they're so near and dear to you—when someone's doing something you don't agree with, it's very easy to point fingers and criticize. At the end of the day, however, we learn over and over again how major this pandemic is and that we just don't have a handle on it. I find myself not being very critical of people right now.

I have this belief that everyone right now is trying to do the right thing, whether they're vaccinated or unvaccinated, or making vaccines mandatory or not mandatory. Then again, I don't have a strong opinion on vaccine policy right now because I don't know what the right answer is. In as much as I'm vaccinated and I believe in getting vaccinated, I won't force people to do it either. I haven't made it mandatory in the bank, although through training and incentive, today 93 percent of our employees are vaccinated. On balance, I'm making testing mandatory and if they don't test, then they get terminated. I'm a lot more comfortable with that approach to safety than the other way around.

Peter Ingram (Hawaiian Airlines) It's the biggest wild card for us. Whether that changes, whether they start to say, "Okay, if you're vaccinated, you don't need to quarantine or you don't need to test," then that's going to change that dynamic. Korea has already apparently communicated that for people who are Korean citizens who travel outside the country after they're vaccinated, they're not going to have to quarantine.

I think that business could come back. What I don't know is whether that's going to be September or October, or is it going to be December or January before that happens? I think the fact we said all year last year, "There's a lot of pent-up demand for travel," and people sort of nodded and kind of believed you, but when we got to January and February and the bookings started taking off like, "Oh yeah, that's what pent-up demand looks like." I think we're going to see that for Japan and Korea as well. *

CHAPTER 7

Lessons Learned

From every crisis there are lessons to be learned. In fact, common sense dictates that those involved in crisis management debrief as to what went well and what could have been done better. The COVID-19 pandemic has not come to end, as everyone had hoped, and there will be a need to debrief once the pandemic is behind us. In the interim, there are some key takeaways that we can talk about.

1. Leadership is important and the ability to make decisions quickly is critical in responding to an ongoing crisis.

Mark Mugiishi (HMSA) I think, in aggregate, we did pretty good. I wouldn't call our response perfect, because we're now trying to overcome the economic obstacles we have to get back to being a vibrant community like we once were. I think we'll take a few years and we may suffer some consequences later because of the debt, the health debt, we created for ourselves. So that's possible, but that being said, we're pretty good. You look at how we did compared to most other places, I would pick us over most places.

Kirk Caldwell Almost everywhere, yeah, in terms of per capita deaths and positive cases.

Mark Mugiishi I wish there was some way for many of the things that I was advocating to move a little faster; they didn't come to fruition quickly, but two months later they happened. If I could have figured out a better way to be convincing, that two months mattered. If things started opening a little earlier, we would have had the same result in terms of the COVID infections, but a quicker response to the economic depression and the accompanying negative health effects (e.g., behavioral health, deferred preventive care, health inequity and disparities) would have saved us from problems later on. So my regret is that I wasn't convincing enough or clear enough at getting people to understand that it is safe once we got to a certain point. Shutting down when we did was absolutely the right thing. Then there was a certain amount of data that suggested we can start relaxing those things, we can do it in this intelligent way, and we can do it now. And I couldn't convince people of that. So I wish maybe there was a better way to communicate that.

It's a once-in-a-generation thing, and for me it was even more interesting because as you know I was a surgeon for most of my life. Then I came to HMSA to pursue this dream of transforming this organization into something that cares about population health and doesn't just pay claims as an insurance company. I got my message out there, got the board onboard, and they said, "You know what? You can run this company and do it like that." And the second they did that, this pandemic hit. As CEO, it was my first real major test as a leader, to navigate this company through the pandemic. So, yes, it's as difficult as anything I've ever done and faced, for sure.

You don't always get an elected leader that can be a good wartime leader, but when you've got a war, you need one. Again, it's something you don't think about much, but don't waste your vote. Always think about when you make a vote, Am I really voting for the right person? and not just the person who graduated from my high school, whatever reason, that kind of thing.

Again, I'm an optimist. This was a generational pandemic and we're going to make it. What I say as an optimist is don't bet against human beings. We fight and squabble, have fits and starts and everything, but, generally speaking, we prevail.

Ray Vara (Hawai'i Pacific Health) In my mind, the most important thing we learned during the pandemic was that leadership matters. It was a time when leaders were required to step up and make decisions.

The good news was that given the nature of the pandemic environment, it allowed us to 1) be nimble, and 2) be humble enough to correct course when necessary. Each day brought a different level of awareness that may instigate a different decision. I saw leaders who were willing to lead and willing to make those adjustments, sometimes on a daily basis.

Kirk Caldwell Look, we opened once and had to shut down. And the second time we did it differently, recognizing that we needed better metrics so that people could understand the consequences of their actions.

Ray Vara I think for the group of leaders who were trying to instigate some of those changes, we had to act on what the most current information was telling us. We also understood that any structures we put in place or decisions we made would be subject to criticism.

David Ige (Governor of Hawai'i) It's about trying to get the right advisors. Trying to make it clear to everybody that we want to have the discussion about what is the right thing to do first and foremost based on the best guidance we can find. Ultimately, it ends up being a policy decision, and I tell the team that I'll take responsibility for that. I don't want them to think about what the political ramifications are and then presenting a recommendation that's filtered by that. It really is about trying to get the best advice first and then think about what it is that we can do to implement.

Kirk Caldwell It doesn't keep you up at night?

David Ige It does keep me up at night. I do recognize that I signed up for the responsibility, and I will take full responsibility. I know that's part of my job. I stay focused on what I believe to be in the best interest of the community and I know that every decision we make is going to make some people unhappy. You just gotta know that as an elected public official, you have to decide how you want to deal with the criticism and all of those kinds of things. I've always felt for all of my time in public service that if you're focused on making the best decision on behalf of the community, all the noise will go away, eventually. As long as you're true to that, to making the decision that is in the best interest of the community, that things will work out in the end.

I still remember going to the new governors conference, the National Governors Association, right after the 2014 election. It was up in Colorado, and sitting governors would come in and have sessions. Governor Jay Nixon of Missouri was in office. He was late to the seminar because he was in Missouri and he just flew in to present. The session was in the middle of the Ferguson riots in Missouri, and he came in and just said, "You guys just gotta be prepared for an emergency from day one, because you never know when it's going to happen. The reality is, as governor, all the best laid plans can disappear in an instant and then your term will be consumed with an emergency." And he talked about his re-election efforts, what he focused on and promised as part of that campaign to get elected, and then Ferguson happened. That whole thing just consumed his entire second term. Dealing with racial inequity and the riots and all of that. He just talked about how that's the job and you can't prepare for it, but you have to be aware and you have to be willing to recognize that the buck stops in the governor's office. You have to be ready, willing, and able to take the actions necessary as governor. That definitely is something that I was prepared for. I didn't anticipate that there would be so many emergencies, but it's something that I knew—I would be in charge and take action, I would have to be willing to make decisions and get criticized for whatever ended up happening.

I'm still proud of the fact that Hawai'i has had better outcomes than any other state in the country. The infection rates up until this last surge were the lowest in the country, our economy is booming again—it's not totally back to pre-pandemic levels, but we are ahead of schedule by everyone's estimates about where our economy would be at this point, and obviously I don't think anybody anticipated that COVID would be with us for so long. Safe Travels worked even better than we had hoped. The economy has responded quicker than anybody had anticipated.

I know that there are critics all around the state who felt like different things should have happened, and I think everybody's entitled to their opinion.

I really don't have any regrets. I know that it's impossible to not get criticized and it's even more challenging in today's social media environment, but I stay anchored to the belief that the public will recognize actions at the appropriate time. If you have to think about what the public comment would be, you'll never be able to make decisions that are necessary.

I know I get criticized for not responding, but it's a no-win situation. I think that's the downside of the technology. Everybody has a megaphone, you can criticize and comment, and the internet provides you a place to hide. If it's a personal discussion, what you would say to me face to face is different than if you can be anonymous. It enables the critics and the deniers the opportunity to be ugly, be the worse that they can in order to advocate for their position. And that's not helpful.

I think that all of the cabinet members, they understand that I want to hear what they would recommend, but at the end of the day they understand that it's my decision and once we make it they are two hundred percent behind implementation.

2. Better decisions are made and more gets done by working together.

Peter Ho (Bank of Hawai'i) There were plenty of times when I said why are we taking so long to do this or that, but fundamentally I understood the reasoning behind it. Part of me was also thinking that the private sector and public sector had never worked so closely together before in our history. It was very interesting to me. You and I know each other, but Scott Saiki (Speaker of the House), I've spent maybe five minutes in my prior life, prior to the House Committee, dealing with Scott, and you come to realize how much of a lack of appreciation we respectively have for the realities of our lives. Scott, he runs the House, he's the leader of the House, he doesn't know what Bank of Hawai'i does on a regular basis. I'm the same way. I work here. I don't know the challenges he has. The one silver lining was the ability to begin to interface around a real problem.

Kirk Caldwell So what lessons have we learned for the future? You are part of Duane Kurisu's core group in terms of his Hawai'i Executive

Collaborative. It's about the public and private sector working together to create/preserve our community, with aloha, while also embracing change, addressing ALICE families living one paycheck away from poverty, and other critical bottom-line issues such as education. And during the pandemic, you were part of the meetings, held with us once a week, that came out of the infrastructure developed by the Collaborative pre-pandemic. It really showed what could happen when the public and private sectors came together to tackle a problem too big for any one sector to solve by itself. It shows how important the Collaborative is for a better Hawaiʻi.

Peter Ho I have a belief that because of our history as a community, that business and government, they just have a naturally adverse relationship. It could be two people with no histories at all together except the history of this side and the history of that side. You don't start out at zero, you start out at minus something. And I hope that maybe through this experience that will change a little bit.

Kirk Caldwell I want to circle back to the food distribution, which for me was one of the most moving things the City participated in. I know you were there at some of them. We were approached by you and Micah for the City and County of Honolulu to participate in this food distribution program. How did that come about? How did you know that people needed food but maybe could not afford to purchase it?

Peter Ho I'm always surprised at how shocked people are about ALICE statistics, when you say more than half of Hawaiʻi's families struggle to make ends meet. Struggle! Like, if they lost their job for a month or had a huge, unexpected expense, their cash flow is completely upside down. So, obviously, when you shut down an economy, I was truly fearful. We know, this is what we do for a living. We know what people's cash flows are like. And you disrupt that for thirty days—we just knew. You're going to have people who don't have anything in their refrigerator.

But when you talk about what happens when someone's paycheck stops coming in for thirty days, or even fourteen days—I know because this is my business, I know exactly what that means. And that's why, thankfully, Micah—Micah's the master at pulling all these different levers. And, thankfully, we knew that you would 1) understand very quickly the dynamics of the situation, and 2) would react, positively, with an action approach whereas others might not. That's how that actually came about.

Ray Vara (Hawai'i Pacific Health) The other thing we saw was a spirit collaboration amongst all sectors of our community in a way that was unprecedented. I hope as a community that we allow that to continue forward well beyond the pandemic. I see indicators that suggest that's going to be the case.

Kirk Caldwell Micah, do you think we're stronger as a community?

Micah Kane No doubt we're better today than we were going into the pandemic, but I don't know if we're going to use what we built. I hope we do.

Georgette Deemer Management changes during the pandemic?

Micah Kane You gotta delegate and you gotta trust. People are a lot stronger. Just a flatter operating model.

Georgette Deemer Will you be changing how you serve the community going forward?

Micah Kane It reaffirmed that we have systemic challenges that are compressing families from thriving in Hawai'i. We started the 2020 legislature with a pretty unified voice. Identifying what we felt were three systemic inequities in our community: access to early childhood education, affordable housing, and a degree of income inequality. We knew we had to increase the revenue side, but no one side is going to solve the problem.

This was the first session (2021 legislative session) we went in where the Chamber of Commerce Hawai'i was actually supporting an incremental increase in the minimum wage. You had both House and Senate and the governor's office unified around an affordable housing strategy and a ten-year early childhood education model. The pandemic just upsided that. I think we were seeing elements of that before the pandemic, but it just reaffirmed that those systems have to change.

Sherry Menor-McNamara (Chamber of Commerce Hawai'i) We've seen a lot of partnerships come out of this. Even competitors helping other competitors. Partnerships, collaboration, and helping the greater community. Businesses were bleeding money but still helping out, donating goods and services. Whether it was for the food banks or other types of organizations and efforts that were in need of products and services, or money for that matter.

3. The feeling that we are all in this together was perhaps stronger in Hawai'i and helped businesses to work more closely and cooperatively with their customers and business associates.

Chris Benjamin (Alexander & Baldwin) Within our occupancy, we lost very, very few tenants. Almost all our tenants survived the pandemic. Business is back in Hawai'i. I'm sad about the ones that didn't make it. We tried to accommodate them as best we could, but as you know for a lot of them rent was just a small part of the equation. The staffing and the other things were too much and some of them couldn't qualify for the Paycheck Protection Program (PPP) or were too late to the game so they couldn't do it.

I'm proud of the way that we, from day one, said, "Look, it's going to be better to work with tenants and have them in place when the pandemic's over than to try to wring every last penny out of them that we can, because then you'll lose them."

Kirk Caldwell Did you have a lot more people working on this?

Chris Benjamin No, I've just got a great group of employees that did this. The thing is, as CEO, it's easy to say I want to work with our tenants, but our team is trained to collect rent, trained to negotiate lease extensions and higher rent, and all that. They had to turn on a dime and change their perspective. And that was not an easy thing.

The way that got executed was Lance Parker, who heads up our real estate group, met every week—maybe every day, certainly multiple times a week—with his top two lieutenants who manage the portfolios, both the leasing side and the property management side. And they would go over every situation that came in so there was consistency in how we handled things. Because a lot can get lost in translation between the CEO and the property manager. But with that system that they put in place, they reviewed every rent relief request so that there was a consistency in how we were implementing it. The property managers were going crazy and they were doing most of it virtually. They had to do it on Zoom and some of them, once they had permission to go back to the centers, they were back there meeting with tenants. Most of it was all done over Zoom and phone calls and it was a challenge. I'm very proud of how they managed that.

Certainly, a pandemic is a very difficult time. I was worried for the safety of my employees, I was worried for the future of my business. But there were other aspects of it that were a little bit easier because some decisions were no-brainers. To send people home, that was an easy decision. I'm not going to put people's lives at stake by having them come into the office, for the sake of what? Even now, a year and a half later, we're still voluntary. You walk through here, there are a lot of empty offices. Nobody's been mandated to come back. So things like that were easy.

Another thing that was easy, that made it somewhat easier, was the fact that we were all in the same boat. You talk to Peter Ingram and think about his revenues down 96 percent. I mean, it's interesting; my revenue is probably down 30 to 40 percent and I'm feeling sorry for myself. And Peter, with all his fixed costs, his revenue's down 96 percent, you start to realize that there are other people who have it worse than you. And then there are businesses where you never would have predicted it, but their revenue just took off. Like Matson is just killing it because they're serving China. But the point I was making is we're all in it together.

4. Hawai'i's consensus nature made our response to COVID-19 unique and different than other places.

Peter Ingram (Hawaiian Airlines) I think to a certain extent that's human nature. It's very much Hawai'i nature, trying to come to that consensus, and I think that has challenged us in the decision-making. At some point, if you're not going to get to a point where everyone's in agreement, at least you've got to make a decision and start moving. It is interesting from the standpoint within the United States, we clearly took, as a community, a more cautious path with COVID than any other state. Even when we were modeling some of the pretravel testing originally, we were talking about modeling after Alaska. Alaska never had the enforcement mechanisms to follow through on that, so it was really a bit of a quarantine with a nod and a wink.

And a testing regime. That was very different here, but if you think about our example internationally, there are people who took an even more conservative approach. Australia and New Zealand in particular. Or American Samoa, where we used to serve regularly, where we'll serve regularly again, but they've taken an approach of trying to completely eliminate the disease, or not have it ever, which they have accomplished but at great emotional cost to some of their people. There are families who have been separated to this day. Fifteen months later, people who were traveling to the Mainland who haven't had a chance to get back to American Samoa.

I don't know that there's necessarily a moment where you can say we got this right or we got this wrong. It was different. And people can come to different judgments about where the right balance is.

5. The federal and state government must stand up a better health posture. Communication was far from perfect and was made more difficult by the politicization of COVID in the final year of the Trump administration.

Peter Ho (Bank of Hawai'i) You know, I have no regrets. Every frustration I felt, I feel I can completely understand at this point. I think that the real issue is what we choose to do from the lessons we learned from here on out. If we don't actually stand up both on a national and local level, a better public health posture, then shame on us. If we don't invest in a better pandemic response infrastructure or disaster infrastructure period, then shame on us. Longer term, if we don't diversify our economy a bit, shame on us.

What happened to lots of well intentioned, good people after this crazy once-in-a-lifetime event, once-in-a-few-lifetimes event, is that stuff happens. And the irony is, you and I both know lots of people who got the decisions right, but boy was it hard to get them to get the decisions right.

Libby Char (Hawai'i DOH) My perspective has changed, it's evolved. It's probably affected by a lot of these things. I don't have a background in public health and I don't think I really appreciated the public health perspective of mission as much as I do now. I have a better understanding of the role of public health and the power of public health, and also the challenges. I didn't really appreciate that before, and I have a much better and more sophisticated appreciation now.

I'm in a position where maybe I can help effectuate some of the change, like having a district health officer for the City and County of Honolulu, and take advantage of some of the lessons we have learned thus far from this ever evolving pandemic. The public health infrastructure was set back by the recession over a dozen years ago and then again by COVID. Let's hope we can begin rebuilding so we end up with a more robust public health system in Hawai'i.

Georgette Deemer One of our leaders said, pre-pandemic, that people in Hawai'i wouldn't have been able to name the director of the DOH to save their lives. But now, you've become the most important person in the state.

Libby Char I think there are a lot of people who are fighting a good fight, but to some extent were overshadowed by all the negative stuff that was going on. They weren't allowed to do what they needed to do. So I think that's one of the things that I've been trying to do is tone down the negative stuff, highlight all the hard work and good effort, and let the smart people who understand public health do their work. It's not so much that it has much to do with me, it's more just letting them have a voice and do what needs to be done. They're the smart guys who know what they're doing, not me. And the team at DOH is working so hard on behalf of all of us.

Georgette Deemer But that's the sign of a good leader. You have good people around you and you let them do their job.

Libby Char And encouraging them. Slowly trying to chip away at that takes a while. We need to change the whole culture and place appropriate value on the importance of a healthy, robust public health system. There are a lot of good people. The bench wasn't as deep as I expected or as robust as I thought it would have been. That was a big eye-opener, and the salaries and stuff at the State, some of them are just dismal. That's been a really big challenge. We need to help the public understand the value of public health so that we prioritize and resource it properly.

There are also a lot of lessons that we learned that I think we're trying to capture now to create strategic planning going forward and a stronger framework and stronger department. We need to pay attention to workforce development, identifying that we should be the best place in town to work if you want to be in public health. What a great place to work—you have access to all of this, this is the mission, this is what's being done in this department. It's so diverse and there is so much opportunity! We are trying to create these partnerships early on with the university, with others, to not only train people but also to do more in the way of internships, training, research, and letting people experience the power of public health. Let's get some grant money and be creative, let's pay public health employees appropriately, make it more attractive, build these bridges now so that we have a better collaboration in training a workforce where they have a job that pays decently. We have work for you to do, it's interesting work, it's fascinating stuff. So we are trying to do some of that now while we can. That's a lesson learned.

Kirk Caldwell You may not be able to match the salary of the private sector, but you can give them a very good work experience, particularly if they want to do public health. DOH could be the place to be. And you can have dramatic impact on a lot of people for what you're doing.

Libby Char And even if you come in and you work for three years or five years and then you go out into private industry, that's okay too. Because at least you have an appreciation for what the DOH does, what the State does, and the role of people and how you tie into private industry and build some collaborative relationships or synergy.

Kirk Caldwell So are you working pretty much seven days a week still? Has it gotten a little better for you?

Libby Char A little bit. The deputy directors of health and the entire leadership team are all just busting their butts. Vaccination is going well. The next big challenge will be reopening schools. That's a huge lift and, thankfully, Dr. Sarah Kemble and her team have really been addressing that. But there is a lot of other stuff that's been put on hold for a year that needs to be tended to. It's only in the past month that I've finally had a chance to start meeting with my dozens of divisions within the DOH.

Kirk Caldwell How large is your employee base?

Libby Char DOH has almost three thousand positions. It encompasses environmental health, behavioral health, public health, and the administration of all of that. It's extremely diverse and my team reminds me that we take care of people from before birth until after their death.

We're trying hard to capture the lessons learned from the pandemic and work on strategic planning going forward. There's such a steep learning curve to working within state government.

David Derauf (Kōkua Kalihi Valley) I think we did the best we could, given what we knew. None of us had been through this before.

We were all misled, too, at all levels of government, we weren't getting great guidance. We didn't have rapid testing available early on, we didn't have good advice, and fortunately we disregarded the advice on masking, so we masked up in Honolulu. Given the limitations of what we knew, we did well. But as I say, I think always we should be asking ourselves *What could we be missing here? Is there another perspective that we need to be listening to?* One thing, I know some smart people who are on the other side of the political spectrum from me, real strong Trump supporters, and I tend to be quite dismissive of their opinions. I'm no longer as dismissive of their opinions. I'm trying to forge, trying to understand them, find out where we have common ground, trying to build bridges there. Because that "othering" has got to go. We've got other challenges coming our way, as we know, like global warming, and we've got to start figuring out how can we get along and how can we do a lot less dividing and a lot more of bringing together.

If there's one thing Hawai'i can teach the rest of the world it's that. We have a chance to be a leader in the world for some of that. Another doctor that Jon Dworkin and I got to know, a very smart infectious disease doctor who worked at Tripler this last year. He's a strong Trump supporter, but you get to talking to him about it and you understand more of what he values: He believes in a business ethic, pulling yourself up by the bootstraps; he believes in getting a good education, doing it on your own—and those are all good values. There's common ground there. In the heat of the moment, I was too certain about my own views on some of this. I'm a lot less certain now. I'm a lot more open-minded.

Sweden is a great example. A close friend who had Sarah Park's job years ago, a smart epidemiologist, he and I for the last eighteen months have had this running argument about Sweden. I said, "Sweden's doing terribly. Look how many deaths they had compared to Norway and Finland." He said, "Yeah but compare them to the rest of Europe. They're doing pretty well. They didn't lock anything down, they kept their schools open, their businesses and economy are still strong." And we would be at each other's throats over this. At the end of a year and a half, he's come towards my way of seeing it and I've come towards his way of seeing it. We are finding much more of a middle ground in saying, "They chose to do this a different way," "They need to acknowledge the mistakes they made," and "Other places need to say they did some of this well."

Kirk Caldwell Per capita, were the deaths in Sweden from COVID lower or higher than the deaths in Germany?

David Derauf Very similar to Germany and France, but much higher than Norway and Finland. I had to acknowledge that Sweden has a much higher immigrant population than either Norway or Finland. Norway has vast resources; they can weather these storms. They've got how many trillions put away in the bank from their oil money; they were smart. It's been an interesting thing for me, to humble myself a little bit about this. A good starting point is to go back to the scientific thing. Science is not about having the answers. Science is about having questions and being willing to question things and constantly refine our knowledge. What did we do? This conversation is a perfect example of that.

6. The counties, or at least the City and County of Honolulu, need a more robust public health component within the administration to advise the city on actions that need to be taken during a pandemic. Because of that void, the mayor created a medical advisory panel that met every-Thursday evening.

David Derauf There are days when the biological illness you're treating is already such a complex and difficult thing to take care of, even in the best of circumstances, and then you realize that you're far from the best of circumstances. That person doesn't have a family member to be there to take them to their appointments; that person is sleeping hard; that person, the language barrier is too much, doesn't have insurance. It can feel overwhelming just to determine how I can do the right thing for this person.

And going to those meetings (the mayor's COVID advisory panel) on Thursday nights, I looked forward to them because we had vigorous conversations and we didn't pretend we had all the answers. We talked about everything, we wrestled with the ideas, we acknowledged that we didn't know stuff. That was important as a process.

Kirk Caldwell I don't think it happened anywhere else in government in this state.

David Derauf We needed more of that. We should figure that out. Members of the community, private individuals, government entities in an open forum where no one gets blamed for saying the wrong thing but encouraged. Everyone's got an opinion here—share it, none of us know the right answer. We need a lot more of that. And it shouldn't be that hard, but I don't think we've practiced that.

Kirk Caldwell We had shut down, the first time, and I think the group was formed as we started to open up again. Opening up parks first for solo exercise, we had discussions on what made sense, what didn't make sense, but we continued to do it following the model that came out of Hopkins: least risky, most risky. By the end of May we opened up everything including bars. I think you were feeling I was rushing too much. Things were overlapping with each other, not this two- to three-week break between each one.

7. When making decisions to fight the pandemic, more thought needs to be given to the unintended consequences of those decisions.

David Derauf Well, you know I've had the chance to reflect on some of that. Number one, we knew then that you had to be accountable in different ways than we did. But even more important than that is the fact that everything you do has unintended consequences. Everything. And if there was one thing I would do differently going back would be to be more deliberate about what might be the unintended consequence if we shut down schools. What's the consequence of having kids out of school for a year and a half? There are real consequences from these decisions, especially for the most vulnerable members of our community.

The well-off kids, my kids weren't going to suffer. My wife could be at home taking care of them. But what if you were a working mom and dad, and your kids were suddenly at home all day long? So we didn't talk enough about what may be the consequences of some of our actions.

And I don't think we thought enough about people's livelihood. How could we support people? What happens when we shut these things off? I mean, even to this day, as a doctor and a public health person, I am wrestling with the fact that globally ten thousand children die of starvation. Every day. And, there's pretty reliable evidence that that number has gone up dramatically because of all the attention being paid to this one virus.

This (COVID) is not the only thing people are dying of. In this community, this is not the most likely cause that people are going to die of. They may be more likely to die of uncontrolled diabetes, coronary artery disease, hypertension, cancer than they are of COVID. And yet, the world became COVID for all of us. And I think that was irresponsible. We really needed to have a sense of perspective. It's understandable why we didn't. An unknown virus, we knew people could die of it, we knew the hospitals could be overwhelmed with it, we had to respond.

I just wish I had had a better sense of what the big picture is. People are going to be afraid to go to the doctor and they are going to stop caring for their diabetes. We had, I only know of one, thankfully, but we did have one death of a child who died when parents were too afraid to go to the hospital. They were afraid of the virus. The child died at home. So if there's one thing I could do differently it would have been to have a larger picture of—to have a sense of perspective about this. At the end of the day, I don't know that we even know how to review the decisions we made, how well we did with it.

8. Governments need to do a better job in communicating with small business and seek its input prior to making decisions that impact small business.

Sherry Menor-McNamara (Chamber of Commerce Hawai'i) No one had a playbook for this. Our role as the voice of business was to advocate for business. We would have done the same thing, we wouldn't have done anything differently. We did what we had with the resources we had. And for us, it wasn't about what's good for the Chamber. Our attention was going to be focused on businesses. Because if we can keep them open, particularly small and local businesses, then they can continue to keep people employed. Jobs. Because that impacts families.

Kirk Caldwell What lessons did you learn from this pandemic, or are still learning? Life lessons?

Sherry Menor-McNamara Communication is critical. Because there was a lack, just to be honest. Communicating to our members and the broader business community. Insuring there's clarity in communications.

9. Working from home can increase productivity.

Dennis Francis (Oahu Publications) I think people in a lot of cases have been more productive. It gives them the flexibility to manage their day. We don't necessarily care what time you get it done, we just need you to get it done. I think our reporting was very strong. It didn't suffer in any way. I was proud of the fact that working from home has worked quite well.

10. Travel restrictions from O'ahu imposed by the other counties should have been reduced in a timelier manner.

Dennis Francis For me, personally, I didn't know anyone who was directly harmed by COVID, but it did impact me in a personal way, as my older brother passed away about two months ago. He had lung cancer and he went through pretty significant cancer treatment with chemotherapy and radiation from basically January to March or April. He didn't have COVID, but Ohio was still very restrictive and I couldn't be with him because he was in the hospital most of the time and they didn't allow visitors, including immediate family. I couldn't be with him when I knew his health was deteriorating, and then he passed away about two weeks after all that treatment. He just died. It wasn't like we knew that was coming even though obviously we knew he was very seriously ill. But for me, long story short, COVID impacted me in that way because I couldn't see him. I couldn't go and say goodbye or spend some time with him.

There are all these tributaries that impacted people in so many ways, like my example. I was pissed. Because of this damn virus, I couldn't go.

Kirk Caldwell I think no one on this planet escaped some impact from COVID. Even when you say Samoa or American Samoa has no cases, but they're impacted because no one can leave and no one can come in. And it's impacted their families, right?

Dennis Francis The biggest mistake that we made as a state was outside your pay grade—the way-too-long delay of allowing Oʻahu folks to travel to the Neighbor Islands without restrictions. So many folks have family members on the Neighbor Islands. And the testing part, if you have four or five kids, that's a lot of money. You just can't do it. That was a mistake. We could have done that four or five months earlier.

Kirk Caldwell After I finished my term as mayor, I visited the Neighbor Islands on multiple occasions and had to test each time. This added additional costs to the trip.

Dennis Francis I know. It was unnecessary and somebody should have stepped up and said enough already. We can always put it back right away if we see that we made a mistake. We had a story in our paper: Samoan families here for six months and they're stuck, run out of money, "Where do we go?"

11. The pandemic accelerated innovation and allowed restaurants to pivot in order to survive.

Paul Yokota (Zippy's) For us, the pandemic created quite a few long-term changes. Before the pandemic, we had planned to implement certain technological changes over a two- to three-year period. All of these changes were introduced in a condensed six- to eight-month period.

Fortunately, we had implemented mobile ordering by late 2019, but customer adoption was initially very slow. Once the pandemic hit, the mobile ordering and payment via the Zippy's app became the hottest thing. As mobile ordering increased, we had to adjust our operations with changes in business patterns.

Our call center hours were also expanded, as many customers preferred not to wait in lines to place their orders. They wanted to order in advance. And as Jason mentioned, our curbside delivery service became popular, so we had to figure out how to deliver orders to the customers' cars. These are all changes that are likely to stay with us.

Kirk Caldwell They did move quickly. I'd stay in my truck and they'd bring out the food. I'd call to order my Zippy's chili on a regular basis and it was so convenient and safe to pick up on my way home. Looking back, is there anything you would have done differently?

Paul Yokota Looking back now, we probably could have moved more quickly to get certain things done. For example, we knew that the plexiglass and the temp checks were needed when we reopened our dine-in operations and we could have started those changes earlier. As we come out of the pandemic, there are still a lot of unknowns. Knowing what I know today, I hope to be responding further ahead of the necessary changes.

12. More support must be given to Hawai'i's public school system during a pandemic. It cannot be expected to operate in a silo.

Christina Kishimoto (Hawai'i DOE) When I talk to my peers, superintendents at the LEA (Local Education Agency) and SEA (State Education Agency), I think everyone worked like we did. This is what was happening, but one of the unfortunate telltale signs is that about 40 percent of district superintendents are changing this year. They're either leaving the profession or they're switching positions and just trying to start up again somewhere else. Headhunters are making a killing right now with the number of superintendents switching jobs.

Superintendent Kishimoto revealed to us that she had challenges with the state legislature and with the Board of Education, not to criticize, but primarily to describe the conditions she and the department worked under in 2020.

Christina Kishimoto The board would meet but I had almost no one-on-one meetings with my board at all. I talked more to you, Kirk, than I did to my own board. And I don't think anybody knows the extreme isolation of the DOE during this time period. We just worked, worked, worked and did what we had to do. At the end of the day, I'm saying that I'm going to transfer, I'm going to pass the baton. I want the kids to be proud of their school system, I don't want them hearing their superintendent complaining about the board or anyone else. But it's the conditions. Those of us who worked under those conditions, there were lots of war stories we shared with each other. How are you? Stay strong. Do this, do that. And lots of teams getting together. That's what saved me and lots of other superintendents this year.

At a legislative hearing, I said to Senator Dela Cruz, "You're giving me nothing out of this legislature for devices, and do you know that if you open up the newspaper for Mississippi today, you know what you're going to see? You're going to see the state superintendent surrounded by her legislature, her board, and business leaders, who all together just rolled out one device for every child, brand new, in the entire state. They had the priority of all the orders from different companies. And we were still meeting about should we buy devices, should we not? They had photos of these hubs where they were giving it to every child in the state. They weren't even asking the child if they needed it. They said, 'We're going to make sure you have a state-of-the-art device.' That's what's on the front page of Mississippi today and here we are sitting here. You're asking me again, 'How much do you need? Why do you need that?'" That context was very different here, but everybody was working hard across states.

Kirk Caldwell I sometimes say that being a mayor, being a governor, it's a very isolating kind of position. At the end of the day, you've gotta make the decision, but I did have support. You really were isolated, you didn't have the legislators' support, you didn't have your own board's support, and you were out there making decisions that no one had ever had to make before on multiple, very difficult issues that had immediate impact on kids, employees, teachers, and others.

Christina Kishimoto I will say, the governor, when I picked up the phone and called him, always answered. Didn't matter where he was. I told him, "You're like my lifeline. I can call you." His staff would always pick up the phone too. I could call communications directly and say, "This is about to happen and I don't want to interrupt the governor, but can you get something ready with my team?" Yes. DOH was also very responsive. I know leadership changed and Bruce Anderson, when he was there—he was kind of ousted from his position—he was there on call too. Department of Human Services, as Kathy Betts came in, she was great to work with. So I had people that I could call, which was great. It's just that the people that should have been most by my side weren't.

Georgette Deemer Are there things that you learned during the pandemic that should be kept going forward? Obviously, your management changes a lot. Not top-down, but delegating responsibility to your very hardworking staff. What kinds of things did you see happening that should stay on?

Christina Kishimoto I still believe in empowerment in decision-making and in teaming, because when you empower your team, you actually get the best out of them. They are part of that decision. I got criticized about why I was empowering the team. I wasn't at three hundred school sites. How could I mandate them to do something when they knew exactly what that meant at that moment for their school? So empowerment is definitely important.

The other is just, as I always tell my team, you do what's best for kids, first and foremost, and then we'll figure out the fallout for that afterwards. And usually when you're doing something that's best for kids, you're actually doing what's right, certainly within reason. We're in education, you're not the healthcare provider, you're not Department of Human Services, you're not the governor, you're not the mayor, we're not making decisions outside of our kuleana, but within our kuleana—we're the educators.

The other thing is when you have an emergency—I think we always know this with emergency management, and I used to deal with emergencies with rooftops and snow and the awful buildings I used to have in Connecticut. Because of a lawsuit, I got lots of money and got to rebuild eleven buildings. So I've done emergency management for a long time, and in that you make it really clear, I'm the decision maker or I've assigned a decision maker to keep things funneled through to ensure safety and consistency. But you also know the difference between emergency management and delegating authority for people to make their own decisions. It's a balance. Don't try to treat everything as part of the emergency when it's not.

I think that's what people didn't see from the outside. They wanted me to direct everything about what a principal did and that's not even possible. Principals are professionals that I relied on and trusted.

13. A pandemic places extra burdens on those working in education, particularly their leaders.

David Lassner (University of Hawai'i) One of the challenges has been the number of people who hold diametrically opposing positions. On the one hand, I get complaints from parents saying, "Your vaccination numbers are great. Why can't my kid get a fully in-person education?" And my next complaint is from a faculty member who is convinced that teaching in person is the greatest risk they can face. We're pretty mixed and hybrid, but that doesn't satisfy some people. And then we have some hard-nosed anti-vaxxers. I got a note from one of our faculty members, and I'm paraphrasing, objecting to our vaccination requirement claiming it is medical experimentation and a violation of the Nuremberg conventions. I'm Jewish and lost relatives in the Holocaust, so getting called a Nazi for trying to protect public health took things pretty far.

I also received objections saying that testing constitutes a violation of religious freedom because "you're inserting something into my orifice." And one claimed that even requiring masks was a violation of religious freedom since "my face was created by God in his image and therefore UH can't make me partially cover my face with a mask."

Georgette Deemer I hope this person isn't a teacher.

David Lassner Sadly, it was a teacher in the health sciences. So that's the kind of challenging division we face—from the expectation of a hundred percent protection from any possibility of infection to visceral and vociferous objection to any mandatory protective measures.

Kirk Caldwell There's also a concern for those people who get double vaccinated and even get the booster shot getting breakthrough COVID. This happened to one of my friends who did everything the government asked him too. And he has long-haul symptoms to boot. And yet he says shaming people who refused to get vaccinated has got to stop. It does not lead to a positive outcome and it just further divides our community. Those who elect to be vaccinated have good reasons to do so, and those who don't, they believe they have good reasons—you can't be the judge.

David Lassner I agree. I saw a television special that assembled a panel of people who objected to vaccination and vaccination mandates. The moderators talked thoughtfully, respectfully, and nonjudgmentally with them for about two hours. They wanted to try to understand who might be able to change someone's mind about vaccination and how. Several of the panelists changed their mind during this two-hour conversation. Others said they would believe their family doctor more than anybody. It was pretty clear that medical guidance could be best appreciated when delivered in person from a trusted source.

Kirk Caldwell Do you think with the FDA full approval of Pfizer that more people will get vaccinated?

David Lassner Yes, when we asked that question almost half of the people who said they don't plan to get vaccinated said a significant factor was the vaccines being under emergency use authorization only. To your point about not shaming people, while I and many believe getting vaccinated was a lot safer than not, we have to recognize that it's not completely unreasonable to be concerned about a vaccine that is not yet fully authorized. Fortunately, that is no longer the case.

Kirk Caldwell Shaming them makes it harder for them to come to the table later. That's the hard part. If you give them respect for what their reason is, they may be willing to reconsider. You're not backing them into a corner. Hard to do sometimes.

David Lassner I've also received nice emails through this. There are people who appreciate how hard a leader's job is in a crisis like this. And many are respectful and thoughtful, even if they disagree.

Kirk Caldwell At the end of the day, you make the final decision. It must be a lonely place to be. But when you say we're not coming back after the spring break and all these kids thinking, I wanted to attend college in person. I want the social engagement with my fellow students and faculty, and the parents want the same thing for their children, and the faculty is evaluating how they are going to be effective teachers if they have to teach by Zoom. So, all of this comes to you, and when you make that decision…

David Lassner You've got to have a team that can share perspectives, ideally, that are different. But when people ask me what's different about this job, I reply that the biggest change is that, ultimately, I have to decide things. As a vice president I could sit in the room and the president would ask what we think and I would be able to share my opinion. Then if it was not a matter in my area of responsibility, I would leave the room and continue on with my day unless asked for more help. As president, I'm now the person who has to assess the input and decide, even when things are murky.

I'm single. M. R. C. Greenwood, my predecessor whom I really like, talked with me about this as she was leaving. Her partner had also been in higher education so M. R. C. would come home and it would be natural to talk about her issues at work. That's a burden on the partner. On the other hand, if you're single you don't have anyone to unload on at home. There are things that I just can't tell anyone.

Tim Cottrell ('Iolani School) It [the pandemic] is not the most difficult thing schools deal with. There are many scenarios that can be considered more extreme. However, it's certainly the hardest, continuous, long period of time where people have to come in and work really hard every day without a break. Typically, schools have a summer break to recuperate, but in order to be prepared we had to use the summer as our time to prepare and plan for the various scenarios that could arise in the coming school year. We recognized that every day potentially presented a new threat or challenge.

Prior to the pandemic, my senior administrative team met once a week for an hour and a half. As soon as this stuff started happening, we started meeting at 8:45 every morning, every day of the week. We'd spend an hour or more together every morning on Zoom reviewing everything and how it affects all constituencies on our campus. While this period of time was very intense, I think it paid off.

Kirk Caldwell And you say the teachers would get time off on a Friday or a Monday. Are you giving yourself time off too? Our senior management team at the City pretty much worked seven days a week during much of the last year of my term. Only in the final months of 2020 did they start to take some time off during the weekends. By then, the case count was coming back down and the early stages of the vaccine rollout were starting to be implemented.

Georgette Deemer Just looking at private schools in general—and I did have an opportunity to talk to Phil Bossert (head of HAIS, the Hawai'i Association of Independent Schools) during that very confusing time period. Are private schools under some kind of protocol situation where you're all kind of doing the same thing or are you free to do whatever you feel is best?

Tim Cottrell The correct explanation of that is private schools like to be called independent schools because we like our independence. No, HAIS has no oversight over us. We ultimately have to follow the rules that the City and State put out. We're not part of the DOE. The DOH can exact influence over us by things that they say, but at the end of the day, we're on our own to make the right decisions and serve our constituencies the best way we can. The checks and balances come into play because of the demands placed on the schools to do well. You can't do anything you want because your parents depend on you and your alumni are watching you. There are many people looking at how you're doing things, but there isn't a governing body that says everybody do this now. HAIS is more of a best practice kind of organization. Everybody gets accredited, so you have to keep your accreditation, but that's every seven years.

Georgette Deemer Well, I can imagine the differences between the really well-funded schools and the independent schools that aren't so well funded.

Tim Cottrell So that's the part that I said was sad to me. All of our materials are open source. Anybody who wanted anything we produced could easily get it online. Our safety plans, protocols, everything—we published, and I think back then when we were making them I circulated them through HAIS to anyone who wanted them. The shame is it didn't take that much. That if you focus on a face mask, a face shield, and washing your hands, that's a long way from a little school saying we can't afford to do this or we can't afford to do that. To me, that's a little bit sad. That somebody didn't come out and say if you can do it this way, it'll work. But that's a risk. In our community, we decided to take that risk, and thank heavens we can say, in retrospect, it worked.

Georgette Deemer Did you get any pushback from parents at all?

Tim Cottrell We've had very little pushback. Our parents were happy with what we were doing online, maybe in comparison to very unhappy parents at other places. So that was fine. When we came back and said it was going to be masks and face shields, we have 3,500 parents or something like that, and maybe two had an issue and questioned why their child was required to wear a mask. Through our consistent messaging with families, we continually stressed how our decisions were grounded in science, and being part of our community meant trusting in these decisions and the guidance provided through credible research and studies. We're like any community. I think we're the only school that's mandating vaccines. So, we mandated vaccines in our upper school. The opposition we get is from the outside world, individuals who are against vaccination.

Georgette Deemer How do you measure the academic achievement in a pandemic year versus a normal year?

Tim Cottrell We were able to do well online and provide all of our students with a nearly normal school year. Our students continued to excel on their AP exams, their SAT tests, and in all other assessments. They all did really, really well. Mainly, just because they had access to uninterrupted education. We didn't really miss a beat there. We also did all we could to support their social and emotional health during this time as well.

We did realize that students coming into ʻIolani for the first time during the pandemic might be behind and we wanted to help. We focused on our entry points, which are kindergarten and sixth through ninth for ʻIolani. We recognized that our students coming into ʻIolani at these entry points may have had a very different academic experience last year, so we added free summer school programs for them to help them prepare. Typically, our summer school courses are around four hundred dollars each. But we offered catch-up courses in math, English, and other subjects so that everyone who was accepted to ʻIolani could take these courses over the summer for free so they could matriculate on a more consistent basis with their peers who went to school here.

Kirk Caldwell Kids who have graduated during the pandemic, what are they going to take out of this? What do you see? What do they write in their yearbooks?

Tim Cottrell There will be a lot more wisdom in retrospect when kids look back and remember what they went through. Kids are incredibly resilient because they go through it and they're not that analytical about it. Instead of *Hey, I wonder what's happening in my life right now?* It's more like *Okay I want to do this today!* So, they soldier on. But I think kids everywhere will probably have a greater appreciation of being with each other. In a world where kind of all the online presence is stressing that for kids, and kids live a pretty healthy life online these days, giving them eight months of only that is sort of like *All right, you're only going to eat ice cream for the next ten months, all you want, and then after that, well okay, vegetables are good too.*

So some of them, I see that. They truly appreciate the time that they have with each other. So you might see when they do reunions twenty years, thirty years, forty years from now, we might see larger groups coming back to be together because they had to go through this.

14. A pandemic tests our trust in government.

Kirk Caldwell You've lived through a lot of crises, but is there anything unique to the pandemic that you learned or that gave you new insight?

Harry Kim (Mayor of Hawai'i County) When I first became mayor, I was asked, "What are your goals?" I said that gaining the trust of the people was my goal, and once gained, I will work every day to keep that trust. Trust is so very important, especially during times of emergencies. It's critical that we have the public's trust.

15. If the pandemic has taught us anything, it is the need for us to become more resilient as a state and as a people.

Ron Mizutani (Hawai'i Foodbank) One thing that I do wish I could have finished was continuing this discussion about resilience and the need for us to have a more… we're not prepared. We're still not prepared. And shame on us if we don't learn our lessons along the way coming out of this. The sad reality is we're still in it. It's hard to implement lessons learned, but in the future I think whoever is leading our state, particularly our state because it's a statewide issue, or even certainly our counties, they need to understand there is a need to focus on food resilience, not so much resiliency. Our infrastructure needs to grow, we need to get our power up and running, all those things are important but without food you're no good. So the plan that I actually submitted to you and your team in the resilience action, that needs to be not only on a piece of paper, that needs to be implemented in an action. It can be adjusted, but that needs to happen. We need to have a food plan in place, we need to have hubs. You know, the food bank is in an inundation zone. That place gets wiped out, we're screwed.

All of that needs to continue, the conversations need to continue, and if it doesn't it will be shame on us. And that's one thing that I would like to do in this role here at PBS. Once this pandemic is pau, continue that conversation and be a vehicle for that conversation to continue. It has to happen. If we get hit by an Iniki on O'ahu, our state will be crippled beyond repair. I honestly believe that.

Kirk Caldwell I agree. It hit a neighbor island and O'ahu was there to help. We had all these resources. But if O'ahu got hit, I don't know if the Neighbor Islands would have enough resources to help us.

Ron Mizutani Not at the ports and certainly not our capacity.

Kirk Caldwell And Neighbor Island people really can rough it. They know how to go out in nature and get things.

Georgette Deemer Do you think that we were the only ones who were doing this kind of integration with our farming community, with our fishing community, the ranchers? Because I don't think I know of any other place that was doing something like that.

Ron Mizutani I can't say that we were the only ones. I do know that some of the Neighbor Islands had a lot more relationships with farmers only because they have more farmers. As far as our brothers and sisters at food banks across the country, we're very different because we're so geographically isolated. They don't run out of produce; they have more produce than they can eat. The reality is they can't send it to us because by the time it gets here it's end of life. As far as being geographically isolated, nobody had to do what we did because it doesn't take that long to get a container of food over. Remember now, besides the fact that we were in line with everybody else to get a can of peaches, what usually took four to six weeks to get here, took three to five months. So we couldn't rely on our food distributors on the Mainland because they didn't have food. And that's why we went to our farmers and that's why we created relationships with our fishermen and that's why we created relationships with our ranchers. The reality is we did not have food to lean on.

Our orders were being canceled by the USDA and everything else. FEMA was in line before us sometimes too. And that's nationwide. So Hawai'i Foodbank was in a real different position than anybody else. Now, were we the only ones doing that? I couldn't answer that.

There were days we looked up and there was no food on the shelves. That probably contributed to my high blood pressure.

Kirk Caldwell I had no idea, when you said it would take three to four weeks to get food and now it takes four to five months at that point. Wow, that is different than everywhere else.

Ron Mizutani We were buying food. Thankfully, we got a head start because we ordered so early in the game. I just told our director of operations, "Just keep buying. I don't care, just keep buying. We don't have money. We'll find the money, just keep buying." We knew that the line was so long to get food and, again, orders were being canceled every day. Meals, stews, chilis, the nonperishables weren't coming in. I'm not kidding you. There was a day when we actually sent our product resourcing director to Costco with a credit card and I said, "Just buy everything you can." We didn't want to tell the community because that would have made everybody panic. I'd go home and drink a bottle of whiskey some nights.

Kirk Caldwell I had no idea, but it makes sense because supply chains were all messed up. That's why you couldn't get things when you needed them.

Ron Mizutani Yeah, it was unlike anything that we ever thought we had a plan for. I'm grateful that people are back at work now and the unemployment rate has improved, but there was two or three months, Mayor, I couldn't sleep at night. I went to bed literally worried about providing food for families, let alone keeping my staff safe and healthy.

Kirk Caldwell I can imagine. Food before anything else. And shelter. The basic necessities weren't there. When you talk about it, I think about how dire it was at the time. Most people probably didn't recognize it, although they did talk about what if container ships didn't show up. How much food would be left to supply people on the each of our islands? And you were living it every day.

16. How we view and manage tourism must change. It is part of a resilience strategy too.

Derek Kawakami Most people don't realize how much they depend on the visitor industry. Whether they like it or not, most people don't realize. And I remind our people we like to think of the visitor industry as hotel workers, some restaurants, but I said, "It's everybody." It is a grocery business. It's the vendors that drive the delivery trucks that work on commissions that sell alcohol to restaurants and grocery stores. I said it is our ability to pay our workers so that they can fix roads. So whether people like the visitor industry or not the reality is that 1) we are dependent on it, and 2) there's ways that we can start to improve people's quality of life by identifying what was some low-hanging fruit.

When you talk to people about their frustrations, it boils down to traffic and housing, and their ability to pay their bills and provide for their families. For traffic, we're looking at improving circulation. So one of the things we did was really put a lot of resources to improve the road conditions. One would be like Kaua'i's Waikīkī, which is along Po'ipū. We're installing a roundabout to improve traffic circulation in the area, we're working with the private sector for shuttle services, we're looking at our parks, looking at implementing nonresident parking fees and having shuttle drop-offs, because we're just trying to provide some pressure valves so that we can also poise the visitor industry. We also had a leg up as far as regulating the vacation rental market. Kaua'i was the first one to really grab the bull by the horns and create an ordinance that basically put a cap on the vacation rentals, saying, "All you guys operating out of the visitor destination area, show us your proof of paying your transient accommodations tax and general excise tax from this date and you are authorized to come in and apply for a certificate. Don't fall out of compliance until you get this thing."

And then the next big step that we had to do was really continue to negotiate with the third-party platforms like Airbnb, VRBO, to get them to understand what it is that we're trying to accomplish and when they finally got it and then settled in, they said, "Well, of course we don't want to be marketing illegal activity." I said, "Well I'm glad that you came to your senses because that's all we're really asking for: use our list of vacation rentals and the ones that aren't on the list, don't let them advertise because you are promoting an illegal activity and that doesn't sit well."

And so you're going to line all those things up and, in a sense, it makes our ability to start to move on some of these improvements much, much easier. It's a lot of work. It just requires a commitment to hold that beat steadfast as far as enforcement goes.

17. A pandemic creates acts of kindness from places you least expect it.

Georgette Deemer Do you have a favorite story out of the pandemic?

Kirk Caldwell For me, it's as simple as at one of our food distributions, a car drives slowly by after picking up pounds of food and there's this little girl—maybe five years old with yellow sunglasses on, her face pressed up against the back seat window of the car she is riding in—and she has a handmade sign with flowers all over it and it says, *Thank you, Mr. Mayor, for the food.* It just made me choke up. It's so sweet. But here's this little girl whose family needs food and she is grateful.

It's those kinds of things. You sometimes don't see the faces of those being impacted by the decisions you are making.

IN SUMMARY, WE THINK MAYOR VICTORINO SAID IT BEST.

Mike Victorino (Mayor of Maui County) I think we've learned one thing. We are part of worldwide, nationwide, and statewide connected communities and unless we work together, we will have more challenges in the future. Hopefully, we've learned from this, with the good Lord's will, to diversify our economy. And finally, Maui will be the community that I believe we are—a resilient, sustainable, considerate, and collaborative group of people willing to step up at any time to help each other out. ✻

CHAPTER 8

Through an Aspirational Lens

Hawai'i is different from every other state in our nation, and perhaps different than any other place in the world. This in part comes from it being the most isolated group of islands from any other landmass on our planet. Hawai'i's uniqueness also comes from the Native Hawaiian host culture that imbues so much of who we are as a people. Overlay that with the strong Asian influence that grew organically from Hawai'i's plantation days, and you get a blend of the most unique group of people living anywhere in the world. This resulted in special outcomes when dealing with the COVID-19 pandemic.

Libby Char (Hawai'i DOH) I think our experience is, in many ways, the same as other places, but I think we have some unique factors. One, just the geography. We're an island state. And so we have this natural border. Second, the counties are all separated and so that's made a difference in terms of things that we're trying to do at a state level. You must take into account that there are significant differences county to county. Third, our cultural background actually lends itself to our population doing a really good job. We have much better mask compliance than many places on the Mainland. And I think some of that is that Asian culture and then the local culture that's adopted a lot of those influences. People in Asia have been wearing masks for years and years. So I think it's more acceptable here.

Politically, I think we're a little more willing to listen to the science. In Hawai'i, I think we still have a sense of "us" and community and that's been tremendously helpful. We see ourselves as having a responsibility for each other. That's a lot of what this is. It's you do things for yourself, but you also do things for your family and you do it for your community. And I think maybe Hawai'i does a good job at that on a state level.

Governor Ige agreed with Libby Char with the caveat that the pandemic laid bare the difficulty the DOH had dealing with the problems of implementing a statewide response to the crisis. Much of the ability to roll out pandemic response programs was better addressed by the counties. Yet, the State of Hawai'i had its own DOH arm to rely on. The other counties did not. They had to improvise with assigned "health officers" from the DOH. It was an imperfect system.

David Ige There are a couple things that are remnants of statehood. There's no other state like Hawai'i. It is the most centralized government in the United States. The State is responsible for public education—there's no place else in the country that does this. The State is responsible for jails—that's a county function in every other jurisdiction. The State is responsible for health—in other jurisdictions, the counties have a public health department.

And so I've had a lot of discussion with Libby, especially since she was on the county side, and the reality is that even though we're given the responsibility for both state and county levels for public health, we're not staffed to be able to respond to the public health emergency. We're not. There probably needs to be either an expansion of the DOH to be able to better support counties or there should be a public health authority at the county level to be able to respond.

If you just think about the mass testing we did. If the State had to try to do that mass testing, we don't have the resources to do it. If it wasn't for the fire department and the county being able to step up, we don't have the people to be able to execute like that. It's the same thing with enforcement. I don't have an enforcement arm, but I'm responsible. So there are a lot of those kinds of remnants of how we're structured that is probably not in the best interests of the community. But to try to change those things is a huge, huge undertaking. Libby's talked about the fact that she thinks we need to have a state health response and a county health response. She said every other state has one and that's why LA County has a health person in charge. So definitely the anomalies in how government is organized in the state of Hawai'i gets exposed in these kinds of emergencies.

Clearly, our DOH is not large enough to be able to handle the statewide responsibility and the counties don't have a health function, which is not the ideal situation. Under normal conditions it probably works okay. In a statewide emergency where every county is dealing with the health emergency, it hampers us in the response.

Micah Kane (Hawai'i Community Foundation) Our lens in Hawai'i has evolved to be one that evaluates the downside of things versus being driven by the upside of something. It's a completely different mentality. Even the pandemic, I think the trick is going to be how we move from a negative lens to an aspirational lens. We don't have muscle memory there. All our muscle memory sits in the negative lens. We evaluate risk, and the structure of how we operate is symptomatic to that, and the moment that risk sits on one of our laps, we lose sight of the aspiration. And until we do that, I don't think we're going to see the kind of Hawai'i that we're capable of being.

Kirk Caldwell Can we change that?

Micah Kane I think we have to. Ultimately, I think it sits in a more civic movement. I believe that.

Kirk Caldwell What's a civic movement?

Micah Kane I think a community that recognizes that they sit in seat one in our political system. Right now I think they've lost trust that their voice has any real impact. For us at Hawai'i Community Foundation (HCF), that whole common data sharing, collective action drives down to how do we get to that mom or that dad or that household to know how their community is performing? So that when they go to the voter box, they have a scorecard in their head on where their leader sits on these issues. And if across the state we're looking at the same data, maybe we've got a better chance of a civic community thinking and vetting their leaders through a common data set so that there's shared goals and maybe a collective action. Right now, I think that communication line and that information line is broken.

Kirk Caldwell Does it have to do with the fact that we have a strong Asian sensibility in terms of aspirations? Thinking big, but don't think too big. Don't dream too big. Don't be *tantaran* (show off, boastful).

Micah Kane I don't think it's any race. I don't think it's racial; it's generational though. I don't know if you've read the book *Five Generations*. There's one generation that makes the sacrifice, they make the ultimate sacrifice. I think of it kind of like the plantation community. They didn't have access to education, they didn't have access to banking, they didn't have access to capital, that was the *tanamoshi* fund? That's how Central Pacific Bank came up, came out of your backyard, Hilo side. That generation made the ultimate sacrifice.

Their next generation, the children, are reminded every day by the moms and dads who made those sacrifices why they're able to get some of the benefits that they've been able to get. Why they can go to school.

The next generation, grandkids of them, maybe we're reminded during the holiday season when they get together for Christmas with grandma and grandpa, and they go, "Eh you see your granfaddah? You know, he wen sacrifice for you. You know, pay respects to him."

And then the next generation comes, and you're dealing with the great-grandparents and they're so far removed. You got fifty kids and then the great-grandparent passes away. And that's the only time that generation hears, "You know what your great-grandfather did in order for you to go to Stanford?" And you come to realize, wow, man, the next generation, you end up becoming what they fought against. You just aren't reminded every day. You don't have those pressures on you. I feel it in my own family. My life is a lot better because of the sacrifices that my dad and mother made, and before that, my grandparents. And my kids, they live really good lives and I'm not sure they know how much their grandparents sacrificed back in the '40s for them.

Until you restart that civic engine again, the question is does it happen during a crisis or does it happen through great leadership? I sure hope it happens through great leadership because the crisis one is painful.

Kirk Caldwell It's hard. We work on it for a while when there's a crisis, and when the crisis goes away, we say that was hard but we're still doing okay.

Micah Kane Senator Inouye had enough juice for many years to make up for that dysfunction, and he was able to call in and force some alignment. That doesn't exist now and I think the power structure got parceled across our community. I don't think there's any one leader that's going to come and do that again. And it has to be a collective of leaders.

Kirk Caldwell By the way, I don't think it's a bad thing that power is diffused around the community as long as you have a linkage.

Micah Kane It artificially held us together. A system is not one person. A system is a bunch of influences coordinating constructively together. I had hoped there was a part of the pandemic that upset the apple cart so much that it would force a reconstruction of that, and I still think that opportunity exists. I think what [House Speaker] Scott Saiki did with the House COVID committee provided an opportunity to do that. I think your willingness to represent the 80-plus percent of our community and to sit in rooms that maybe otherwise was difficult because of politics, and to step over that—you really call it out. It's all our egos that stop us from doing what we need to do.

Kirk Caldwell I think the revolution of 1954, the election of Governor Burns, the early days of statehood, they laid an infrastructure that made Hawai'i a much better place for everybody. So much of it came out of the war and the 442nd and the 100th. Their shared experience on the battlefield—which we can't even begin to imagine how horrific it was, the battles they fought—but also their shared experience coming from the plantation and the prejudice they felt and the opportunity. After all of that, after the horrific experience of war, they said, "We're not going to let this pass. We're going to do something about it." And they did, over two decades. Najo Yoshinaga and those kind of guys, they implemented prepaid healthcare and other things. But it took the legacy of the plantation and a war.

That was a community and there was a trust in government. I think people thought this group could make a difference and they did, so they remained engaged.

Micah Kane That's the word you brought up, trust. I think the other piece of that conversation is this Hawaiian renaissance. You were willing to be at the table on a lot of it. Whether it was the wind farms or the Waimānalo park. It's hard to not acknowledge that as another complexity of this time. I think of that as well as the wrong lens. Our host culture is a competitive advantage for this place. It's not a hindrance. We have to embrace it whether it's how we approach the development in dealing with *'iwi* or trying to bring innovative technology through wind farms and TMT (Thirty Meter Telescope). I often wonder, those things would go, but they would go differently. I think we have to find a way to embrace it.

It has to move from a transactional conversation—all these things are transactional right now, both sides: *What do I have to give up to get? What do I gotta get to give up?* As opposed to, *How do we come to the table? What resources do you bring? What are we trying to achieve?* That to me is shifting from a negative lens to a positive lens. Until we do that, we'll never achieve what we're capable of achieving.

Kirk Caldwell I agree. I think Native Hawaiians need to be front and center in the conversation, in almost every conversation, because that does define who we are, no matter who we are. But I do think it has to be through some form of infrastructure. You mention wind farms. If somehow you allowed all energy generated from wind, sun, geothermal, tides and you form some kind of Hawaiian corporation that got a portion of that revenue like the Maori, if they had a share in revenue, then they have a voice on the projects. And instead of fighting them, they are actually saying we are interested in doing this in a proper way. Astronomy too, I'd put it in there. We have some of the greatest astronomers. So how do we provide them the platform to make the decisions?

Micah Kane Having worked at Department of Hawaiian Home Lands and Kamehameha Schools, that perspective has evolved to one that I think we have to have a culture of a place. That to me is the solution. It can't just be a culture of a single race. If you look ten generations of a Hawaiian marrying outside their race, that generation is .00133 of 1 percent. Of 1 percent! So are you going to expect that *de minimis* part of what makes you who you are carry the culture of this place? To me, it was that culture that was special, how they cared for this place, and that's something that every person that comes here should have a responsibility for.

Kirk Caldwell And some actually take it on.

Micah Kane Yes, they do. And to exclude them from being responsible for that? So when you start divvying up resources, it should be who's committed to the culture being here and how we're going to function. And if you commit to that, then you share in the resources that you started to outline, whether you came five generations ago or fifty generations ago. Because a thousand generations from now, that forty-five-generation difference is nothing, if we believe this place is going to be around a thousand generations from now.

So anytime we take an action like that we're cementing in a system that in the not so distant future it's going to be that much more difficult to break. My whole career has been involved in trying to reconcile what has happened to the Hawaiian people. I'm super passionate about that. Most of my thinking has been around that lately.

Dwayne Steele, who funded ʻAha Pūnana Leo, was one of the earliest advocates for the renaissance of the Hawaiian language. If there was one person I wish I could have gotten to know, it would have been Dwayne Steele. I've heard so many wonderful stories about that man. That's one person I'd want to have lunch with.

Kirk Caldwell He was a developer with Grace Pacific. Spoke fluent Hawaiian. Grew up in Colorado, not Hawai'i.

Micah Kane I don't think any Hawaiian, as we define it today, would not welcome him into their 'ohana. Puakea Nogelmeier is another one. Just amazing aloha spirit.

Kirk Caldwell Looking back, is there anything you would have done differently?

Micah Kane I guess the only thing would be what could we have done to set the table to make sure we don't lose to atrophy? The muscle we built has got to get better, not atrophy. I'm feeling that pressure right now to fall back to what we were. I thought we built some really good muscle—communication muscle, coordination muscle. We reduced our egos, we sat at the table. People that weren't willing to sit at the table together were willing to sit at the table. Both of our biggest banks were major players. First Hawaiian Bank put up a million dollars. Partnering with the University of Hawai'i, they focused on the kids that lost their last semester of education. Those kinds of things, I feel like we can't lose it.

Kirk Caldwell You've got the Hawai'i Executive Collaborative still going strong. There is still a crisis and it's our economy, it's our housing, homeless. I think of all the things we tried to do during my eight years in office to develop more affordable housing, ADUs (accessory dwelling units). There are 120,000 parcels that could have ADUs but there are only a thousand, at a time when we need to build twenty-five thousand new homes.

Micah Kane Look at D. R. Horton. Horton's building every unit ADU compliant, eleven thousand units that you'll get over time.

Kirk Caldwell We passed legislation, Bill 7, Marshall Hung's plan, all affordable rental units—whatever it is we've done, it's nowhere near enough. So you know this muscle that's around the table, government, the private sector, if we're going to be a fair place for everybody, there has to be housing for everybody. And we're not building it.

Micah Kane If I was to say, some of the big accomplishments of your administration are going to go unrecognized, probably the biggest, a lot around the sewer federal decree, and I do think one of the shining stars that went unrecognized is Lori Kahikina. I hope she sticks it out at HART, because I do think she's a solid, ethical, strong, capable leader.

The pandemic also accelerated innovation for businesses and educational institutions in Hawai'i, including working from home or learning virtually.

Georgette Deemer Given your business as a leading bank in Hawai'i, I've started to notice that some of your services have changed, like your contactless cards. Is that a result of the pandemic or were you headed in that direction anyway?

Peter Ho (Bank of Hawai'i) Yes, we were headed in that direction. So we've been heading towards digitization and more digital ways of doing things for a long time. The pandemic accelerated that. So the belief is that the pandemic accelerated the digital transformation and adoption by more than five years—in just one year it leapfrogged. We saw traditional branch traffic fall to half during the pandemic and it's come back a little bit, but not anywhere near what you would expect.

Digitization is a big issue that actually played well to where we're taking the bank, but this work-from-home thing is fascinating. I can't tell you how it's going to play out.

I can tell you that people have gotten very used to working from home. We do these focus groups. Actually, we were ready to tell people, "You've gotta be back by this day," but before we did that, we said, "Let's do these focus groups." And the focus groups were amazing. When you talk about work from home, everyone's so happy about that.

When you're talking about returning to the office—I wasn't in any of the groups, but I'm told their face, their complexion, just completely changed. They don't want to change. So we're in the process of figuring out how the workplace changes permanently. And basically what I've concluded is clearly there've been lots of benefits unlocked by having two-thirds of the workforce working from home, mostly for our employees. They can be home, they can be with their family, all these things. And clearly, there are things that are better, certain functions, when you're in the office. And we're going to be somewhere in the middle. And we're going to try as much as we can to support this side, but we've got real needs on this side. That deal is yet to be finalized, but it's a rocket situation. People, they've found nirvana—it's like waking up, brushing their teeth, not having to jump in their cars or get on the bus.

David Lassner (University of Hawai'i) Do you know Herb Lee of the Pacific America Foundation? He asked me to do an 'Ōlelo show with him called *Silver Linings* that would focus on the positive outcomes, the silver linings, coming out of the pandemic. For one, all of our faculty and all of our students know how to use online tools for teaching and learning now.

We also provided ways to do nearly all our routine business online. I don't sign many pieces of paper for transactions at all anymore. We moved a lot of our approvals to online transactional systems using some good tools we embraced for that. For communications like memos where people want to see a signature, we can paste them in electronically with the right tools. We beefed up our IT security for people to work from home since for some of our systems we need to be very careful about who gets in from where.

I mostly worked from home, but I was coming in about once a week, often to sign things. By the end, I was mostly signing things like retirement certificates and donor thank-you letters that we really want to be personal.

I think one of the biggest silver linings will be the shift to much more online learning. Once everyone understands what's possible, they're much more open to whole degree programs online, which can really create opportunity throughout the state.

Georgette Deemer It might even help your parking problem.

David Lassner We've talked about that. A major aspect of going to college for eighteen- to twenty-two-year-olds is the experience of being on campus, the relationships with other people, the living in a dorm, working in a research lab with faculty. So there's a whole lot of it that's not just about the class. Fully online education tends not to be that effective for eighteen- to twenty-two-year-olds, the prototypical traditional student. We've looked at some of our data on this and what we found is that freshmen actually do well if they take one online class a semester. But if they take more than one online class, their academic performance actually declines. They are less likely to persist in higher education, we think, because they're not as engaged. Fully online learning takes more discipline. As the DOE found, this can be a challenge. You send a student home with a week of homework and they might not do it. Or maybe they look at it the day before it's due. We have to pay attention to the same issues with college students.

That said, online learning is fantastic for adults. They tend to have more constraints of schedule and location that make it difficult or impossible to go to campus during the day. We're going to do much more to provide online programs that are workforce-oriented. Similar to the Oʻahu Back to Work project we did with you, we're doing a second version with the new mayor.

Kirk Caldwell I'm really glad to see it's continuing. On online learning, for some kids in more rural areas, maybe other islands, it gives them a chance to get a college education with not a lot of cost impact or family impact. So you're in Kaʻū and you're also working, it gives them opportunity that may not be there.

David Lassner Yes, no question. And if you're somewhere like Hāna, there are very few classes that are physically offered since the population is so small and we don't have the scale. So there's a whole lot that we can do online to serve them. We need to match the right curricula with the right modality for our students, including much more online for adults.

Georgette Deemer Even back when I was in Nebraska fifty years ago, they were already starting to talk about tele-education because they had a lot of farm kids.

David Lassner That's actually what got me here. I was a grad student at Illinois and I worked in the lab that had developed what was the leading system for using computers in teaching and learning in the '70s. Fudge (Dr. Fujio) Matsuda was the UH president, an MIT engineering graduate, and he decided computers are going to make a difference in education. So he sent a team from UH around the country to visit all the leading places that were working with computers and education. When they returned, UH decided to start a pilot project here that included use of the system I worked with in Illinois, called PLATO. They decided they needed somebody cheap to help UH get started, so I was recruited to come to UH for a one-year, halftime contract in 1977. And I never went back.

Of course, there can be other types of drawbacks to virtual meetings.

Georgette Deemer I know that elections and campaigns are so dependent on media to get their message out, but because of COVID, everybody had to campaign completely differently this time. How did that impact your paper?

Dennis Francis (Oahu Publications) That's a good question. All the virtual meetings were interesting. You can still get the words and the points that candidates are making, but the thing that's always missing is body language—how you deliver your comments and the confidence you show with body language. With virtual meetings, you're only getting a head shot and you don't know what they're doing. Are they reading their comments? You don't know, you can't see. Being in the same room, it's different. You can have a few minutes of small talk. It's not as sterile. Even to this day, these virtual meetings are the one thing that I hope go away.

Virtual press conferences and interviews didn't allow us a lot of time to get a good feel for the person. You clearly get their campaign talking points, but you just don't get that vibe of human contact. You can see how they react on camera, but it's different. Being in the same room can take people out of their comfort zone. And that's how you measure people: how they react to that.

Sherry Menor-McNamara (Chamber of Commerce Hawai'i) I think it forced many businesses to think differently and to ensure they incorporate technology. That's another thing. Many of them didn't have e-commerce sites or any level of knowledge regarding technology and how to integrate that into their business. So, moving forward, I'm sure we're going to see more of that.

Gary Kurokawa (City and County of Honolulu) I saw a lot of restaurants, they said doing takeout was great. They learned that in the takeout business, you could still make money and anyway, you don't need this whole space to be indoor dining. Staffing, all that costs money, so people adjusted.

Kirk Caldwell That's the good and the bad of the pandemic on the labor side. I think as we return, and maybe return to 100 percent despite the economy, there's going to be less workers there. They've learned during the pandemic to get more done with fewer people, because you couldn't have the people, through technology or through changing their systems or techniques.

Gary Kurokawa And then, downtown office space. People learned how to work from home and can take advantage. Some organizations that didn't before can now take advantage of doing with less office space.

Sherry Menor-McNamara (Chamber of Commerce Hawai'i) It's the hybrid thing we've been hearing about. And I think we'll see many who were employed in the service industry pivot to other types of jobs because they recognize *Hey, maybe I don't want to do this.* They want to get re-skilled or retrained or upskilled for different types of jobs. So there's been a lot of moving around.

Georgette Deemer Jason, was anything changed in terms of your relationship with other restaurants? They're your competitors, but in a situation like this it seemed as though the restaurants were rallying more than ever before to get through this.

Jason Higa (Zippy's) That's a great question because what I observed during the pandemic was the Hawai'i Chamber of Commerce working with Hawai'i Restaurant Association, Hawaii Food Industry Association, Retail Merchants of Hawaii. All of these organizations came together because there was a common need. So retail, restaurant, manufacturing, it didn't matter. Everyone was suffering. To her credit, Sherry Menor-McNamara, our president, took the lead in doing things very differently. She implemented significant changes that I expect will continue post-pandemic.

Georgette Deemer It must have been sad because a lot of restaurants had to die and they're probably not going to come back.

Paul Yokota (Zippy's) We're very fortunate to have diverse skill sets as a larger company. Smaller operators may not have all the resources we have, so when they asked for our help with information like our protocol for employee wellness checks in the morning, we openly shared what we were doing. Whenever we were asked, we shared. And other restaurant operators shared with us, too.

Jason Higa I don't know if you know what Denise Yamaguchi did with her Hawai'i Food and Wine Festival organization. The annual Hawai'i Food and Wine Festival was eventually held on a much smaller scale in 2020 and 2021, but Denise really shifted her resources to create the Food-A-Go-Go website during the pandemic. Denise wanted to support local agriculture and she knew that the best way to do so was to support local restaurants, especially the smaller operators. The Food-A-Go-Go website was the means for Denise to support literally hundreds of local restaurants by providing a valuable resource for customers to know who was open and their hours of operation.

Kirk Caldwell She came in and we supported it, but I don't think we did enough.

Jason Higa Denise also assisted these small restaurants by making sure that they applied for their PPP loans. She contacted all the mom-and-pop operators to let them know about the PPP loan opportunity. Many had no idea what to do or how to apply for the PPP loan. So they were encouraged to call their banker and find out how to apply for the PPP loan. Denise did something pretty incredible with creating Food-A-Go-Go and communicating with so many mom-and-pop operators during the pandemic.

Paul Yokota My career started in hotels and now I'm in the restaurant industry. As an island state, we have to think very differently to get things done. For instance, when I worked on the Mainland, you could source inventory from everywhere. If you couldn't get it from one distributor, you could from someone else and it could be trucked in. Not so much in Hawai'i. During the pandemic, we had to be very aware of what we could and couldn't source. We had to be aware of alternative products for substitutions and we relied upon our suppliers for assistance. We had to be reactive at times, but we also had to strategize for the future.

Business survival during the pandemic is not a sprint or a marathon, but more like a triathlon. In the initial stage of the Ironman, you're in the water just trying not to drown, and that's what we were doing. The second stage is cycling, and it's a long stage and covers the most miles but you have the bike. You have tools like the PPP loan to help get you through. With these tools, you can move faster towards recovery. Not everything is going to work, but you can go fast. It's also about positioning in this phase. The third and last part is where we are now, the marathon stage. It's feet on pavement. It's all about guts and discipline and stamina because you're worn out and exhausted, but you're going to get it done and cross that finish line.

Jason Higa I reflect back on how Duane Kurisu leveraged the Hawai'i Executive Collaborative (HEC) to assist the State of Hawai'i during the pandemic. HEC supported the TRUE Initiative, served as an accelerator for ClimbHI Bridge and Movers and Shakas, created the AlohaSafe Alert app, and supported the Hawai'i COVID Collaborative and COVID Pau. Many residents likely have no idea how much HEC contributed to Hawai'i through these many programs during the pandemic.

With Movers and Shakas, we worked directly with the hotels and airlines to support the program, but the advisory board was comprised of organizations without a direct stake in promoting remote workers coming to Hawai'i. No one on the advisory board is benefiting. In fact, all of us contributed resources and money to get Movers and Shakas off the ground. It was all with the hope that maybe we could do something beneficial for the state of Hawai'i.

Kirk Caldwell My hope is that this approach is an example of Biden's Build Back Better Plan where we will grow in a more resilient way. Because it's about bringing in lost and new talent from outside the state and interfacing with our agricultural industry and schools, for example. This could take us in a new direction, a forward leaning direction. Different than before the pandemic. And it's even about tourism. Not where you come and lie in the sun or surf or shop. It's to come and enjoy our community and interface with agriculture and youth and things like that.

Jason Higa Hawai'i Tourism Authority (HTA) recently introduced the Malama program. So HTA is thinking along the same lines and we've been communicating with them about how the Movers and Shakas program could also be a model for changing how our visitors interact with our community. It's creating a different type of visitor. Instead of staying for one week, visitors can remain for weeks while giving back to the local community. And they can do this because they are working remotely while in Hawai'i.

HOW THE PANDEMIC CHANGED THE HAWAI'I HEALTH INDUSTRY

Mark Mugiishi (HMSA) Historically, HMSA is a very hierarchical place for many or most of the decisions were made from the top level. The CEO says something, maybe he delegates a little bit to the senior executives. Well, when this happened, you can't do that. It's all hands on deck. There's too much going on, right? There's trying to assess what's happening in the rest of the world, what are the best practices, what are the federal mandates coming in, what do we need to do to take care of our employers, what do we need to do take care of our members—so everything's changing.

So we created a COVID-19 task force with about twenty leaders at the intermediate management level led by Dr. Stefanie Park, who's our assistant VP of medical management, so not even a senior executive, and surrounded her with a team of leaders at a similar level. And we said, "We're delegating this to you. You guys tell us how are we supposed to manage COVID across the community in every aspect," and they were amazing. They worked tirelessly day and night and everything, in all components. That's new. So now we have an organization where there's an empowered middle management and that will persist into the future. That's one really important thing.

Virtual is another important thing. I'm concerned that we don't go overboard with virtual, but there are tons of advantages in virtual, including the delivery of healthcare. Doctors got comfortable delivering care virtually and patients got comfortable receiving care virtually. It will improve access, especially in rural areas, places where you don't have access to a specific specialist. Now you can through virtual care. Virtual meetings can become more common, so it becomes a little easier to have meetings. The careful thing about that is too many like that and you stifle innovation to some degree. You know how many times we've all been in meetings and people don't say anything necessarily but at the end of the meeting they'll walk up to you and go, "You know what would be a good idea?" And that's when the light goes on and you go, "Oh god, we gotta do that!" That doesn't happen on a Zoom meeting, so there's a balance to that. But I think all those things will forever change a little bit about the way we do business.

And I think viewing at the very highest level, viewing ourselves to the employee level as more than just an insurer came out of this. Because in this thing, we were helping with the mass vaccination centers. We're helping to set policy on how the DOH might create the pillars of health, right? All of those kinds of things. Our employees started saying, "Hey, we're not just here to pay claims. We're actually here to influence the health of the state."

Georgette Deemer So given that you see the doctor/patient relationship also going more virtual, going forward, is that going to change it from an insurance point of view?

Mark Mugiishi Yes, it will change, but there will be challenges. There has to be, right? So the way we cover virtual visits, the way they overlap between a virtual and an in-person visit—obviously, if you do the same thing in both ways you can't pay for it twice. The other thing that the pandemic did, by the way, is that it made the issue of affordability a much more urgent issue. Healthcare was always getting to the unaffordable phase. We spend almost 20 percent of our GDP on healthcare in our country, which is really ridiculous. Way too much. The next closest first world country is about nine or ten, so we're spending double.

Kirk Caldwell What is that country? The next closest country?

Mark Mugiishi Sweden, UK, they're all around there. Canada. Most of them cluster around the 10 percent level, and we're closer to the 20 percent level, and it's unaffordable, right? So that was always a problem and now when there's less money in the world, unless the federal government decides to print more—which kind of makes it less money anyway right, because it's more money that's worth less—it becomes more of an issue. So we continue to put more stress on the economic system by saying that we're going to demand that more and more and more money go toward healthcare. That affordability issue is a big deal. So smarter, better ways to make sure people get the care that they want and have access to it, and affordability are a critical next mission.

Ray Vara (Hawai'i Pacific Health) We said very early on that we weren't going to use the term "new normal." We believe "new normal" symbolizes that the future resembles the old normal. We at Hawai'i Pacific Health (HPH) refer to the future state as Hawai'i Pacific Health Beyond. We quickly developed a plan of what we wanted the future to look like for HPH when we emerge from the pandemic.

The HEC is a 501(c)(3) nonprofit organization created by Duane Kurisu in 2019 to bring together a group of leaders from the private and public sectors throughout the state of Hawai'i to drive collective action to address Hawai'i's most difficult challenges. The Collaborative started meeting approximately two years before the COVID-19 pandemic struck Hawai'i. Through its efforts, it cultivated leadership that is dedicated to the care and nurturing of Hawai'i's land and its people. The community muscle that was developed as a result of these early efforts provided a forum and a platform by which diverse groups and sometimes competing interests were brought together to address various issues caused by the pandemic.

Mark Mugiishi (HMSA) The reason why that collaborative (HEC) was so successful, I think, was because prior to the pandemic all of us had built relationships in person, breaking bread at a dinner table, sharing stories, and feeling connected to each other. And so when this happened, even when we're now connecting only virtually, there's trust, there's understanding, there's belief in each other. I do worry that now that people have found it easy to connect on Zoom or Webex or whatever, if that becomes the only norm, it's going to be hard to build those things for the next generation from scratch. Yes, we'll forever have a virtual meeting as one way of communication, but it cannot ever become the only way. As we look for how we move into the new world, it's going to be a hybrid because I don't believe you can only work virtually and have the same kinds of trusting relationships.

Kirk Caldwell I think there's something to breaking bread. Literally, breaking bread and telling stories to each other and spending some time outside of serious work. Getting to understand each other so you know who they are.

Mark Mugiishi And another place where this happened clearly was in California. Blue Shield of California, which is our sister plan there, early on, they got involved with making sure there was more testing available and they got so close to the governor and the state health department there because of their success at helping them. When the vaccines came out, the State literally designated the whole vaccine effort to Blue Shield of California. They said, "You guys are in charge. You vaccinate our state please." And so part of that allowed them to go from worst to first. At one point they were the worst state in the nation for the percentage of people who were infected, for their positivity rate, everything. Now they're down to like nothing, and they have the highest vaccination rate because they got Blue Shield to vaccinate their state basically.

HOW THE PANDEMIC CHANGED THE BUSINESS COMMUNITY

Chris Benjamin (Alexander & Baldwin) The hardest days of my career were at HC&S (Hawaiian Commercial & Sugar Co.), when I was running the plantation. It was just brutal. In that, I felt like my team and I were in that alone. We were the last man standing in the industry and that was really tough. COVID, I'm not in any way saying it was fun, but there was a lot more company—you knew we were all in it together. And that helped.

Frankly, going through it in Hawai'i was unique because of the island nature of it and we truly were all in it together. Our markets,

Peter Ingram's market, Peter Ho's market, Bob Harrison's market, Ray Vara's market, it's all Hawai'i. These aren't guys who have ten different markets that they're worried about. We're all focused on how do we get Hawai'i through this and get our companies through this? So in that sense it was—let me just say, it could have been worse.

Georgette Deemer I was struck by your comment about being the right person to have to do this deed (closing the last sugar plantation on Maui and in the state) because obviously people understood who you were, and I think the same thing applies in the pandemic situation too. I mean, I can't imagine that a similar corporation on the Mainland would have that kind of sensibility about their tenants and caring about them being there on the other side of this whole thing.

Chris Benjamin Well for better or worse, about four years ago, I came up with a tagline for Alexander & Baldwin: partners for Hawai'i. And when I say for better or worse, I've had people use it against me. I had a tenant call me and say, "Well you say you're partners for Hawai'i, then why are you charging me rent?" Well that's not really how it works. But the good aspect of that is it grounds us and it reminds us if we're going to be true to that, we have to take that approach. We have to take the approach of maybe collecting a little less rent during the pandemic or a lot less rent during the pandemic but having tenants on the other side. And look, it was a happy coincidence that the right thing for the community in my mind also was the right thing for business. Because now all of those tenants are open and they're busier than they were in 2019. Not all of them, but many of our tenants are already exceeding their 2019 revenue. So business is back.

Kirk Caldwell Bob, you talk about all this interweaving, and I was thinking the HEC maybe brought it all together. We have developed a certain muscle in our community. Both private and public sectors working together maybe for the first time in a long time. Could it change us as a community long term? How do we keep this going or will it slowly fall apart as more visitors come and we all start having our own individual problems?

Bob Harrison (First Hawaiian Bank) Personally, I think it will stay with us as long as most of the same actors are there. What we need to work hard for is when we grow out of the current crop of people who went through this together, how do we make sure that as new people come on board due to the natural movement of leaders—not just in the business community, but in government and healthcare too? How do we make sure the next ones don't forget how important this was, this lesson? It will last a little bit longer because the people who presumably will step into the leadership positions will have had some exposure to it, but it's easy to lose.

Kirk Caldwell For me, as the former mayor and someone who cares about the community, keeping it is critical. For me as a government leader, I did not reach out to the private sector, but the private sector reached out to me, a big component of the private sector, and it was for the better. And they did it to the governor and the other mayors. So now you have government and business working together on things that are important for the community, for their businesses. That's the part that I hope continues.

Bob Harrison I think that willingness to be open, honest, and transparent when things aren't being recorded and have honest conversations. There are some things government is meant to lead. Natural disasters are one of them. We look to government for the experts. Public health has been underinvested from a healthcare perspective for decades, and we too often deal with the follow-on effects after people get sick and not the causes. That's the root of our healthcare system, quite frankly, so I think there's cause for re-examination of that. But in a health-related pandemic, people are going to look first to, as we should, the DOH, elected leaders, experts within that industry, and all the follow-on effects.

What we missed this time is that it didn't happen quick enough, and I think there weren't enough outside voices added to that room that were valuable. They made it better. People were willing to invest in the middle of this to do it right.

Ray Vara pushing very actively on more testing, Jill Green doing a negative pressure floor, all that. Ray had cleared out a whole area over here in anticipation of a lot worse outcome. That took foresight, money, and conviction to do it. It would have been nicer to have all that tighter together and that's what we need to learn for next time. That's not something business can tell government to do, because government is in charge. But I think next time we'll be much more proactive in saying, "Hey by the way, these people are really smart and they can help solve this problem for you. You gotta decide, but they can help."

Kirk Caldwell My conclusion, at least with our state health department, is in an emergency, in a hurricane, like you said, people know what to do. But our health department is not wired in any way from the foundation up to respond quickly to a crisis. They're well-meaning people. They're smart; they're doctors, scientists. But they cannot be running the response.

Bob Harrison I think part of that is because it's traditionally part of the National Guard in a disaster. The military steps in, the military system kicks in, but again, we need to do it different next time.

The other thing, even before Governor Neil Abercrombie, I got sucked in this group and Mike Mohr (managing director of The Omidyar Group) got involved in transforming Hawai'i government and trying to get more technology in state government. Primarily, the focus is the State because the City had done quite a bit, but there's a whole bunch of stuff that needs to get done. Look at our unemployment system. Talk about exposing things that need attention. We kicked the can down the road on this and many other technology projects that would have enabled us to move a lot quicker. We did the same thing at First Hawaiian Bank internally. We started doing our PPP loans on paper—it was a nightmare. While we had our software engineers developing a portal to do it, paper was the immediate solution, so a third of the loans got done on paper and two-thirds of it got done through a portal, which was beautiful. It took two and a half weeks to get the portal up, which was a race to the money because we thought the Small Business Administration money was going to run out. Similarly, the State just didn't have the capacity, the capability to handle the volume of unemployment claims.

The lesson learned on this: It's at your peril not to invest in that critical infrastructure that includes technology, because when disaster happens it makes all the difference. Think of the frustration people went through, the people that didn't stay employed and were trying to make legitimate unemployment claims. But that was a huge lesson learned.

Kirk Caldwell to Ray Vara I don't know if you'd agree with this, Ray, but I think we're different than probably everywhere else in the United States. We came together as a community, private and public, working together and I don't know if that was the same in New York or New Jersey or California. I do think that we acted differently in that way, and while we have that big ocean out there that's a real barrier, I think we could have had a much worse situation, and we have limited resources to deal with a worse situation. But coming together as a community early through the leadership that you and your group brought to the table, I think made us very different.

Ray Vara (Hawai'i Pacific Health) That leadership group was a broad set of individuals and they were very impactful for the betterment of Hawai'i.

Kirk Caldwell It is broad, but I think there is a nucleus. We are where we are today because of that group.

Ray Vara I absolutely agree.

Kirk Caldwell I think that's partly why visitors are coming here. They may be frustrated by having to upload and get their QR code, but they're coming here because this is a safe place. *If I'm going to travel, I want to go to Hawai'i.*

Ray Vara I'm very proud of our state. I think that we saw a different side of human nature. We saw people greeting each other on the streets—they were out for walks, you couldn't buy a bike without being on a wait list. All those things I guess were happening all over the country, but I think Hawai'i's experience of those things was relatively unique because of the heart of our people and our geographic isolation. We were in it together.

Gary Kurokawa (City and County of Honolulu) Observing the whole process that we all went through, the determination and the persistency that you guys showed in those meetings, which weren't always positive meetings, from the health point of view, I would think it would have been frustrating at times because government was moving slow. But I gotta say that not once in those meetings did I see you guys being disappointed or discouraged. We would meet again and you guys would be right there with the message. You guys are trying to move everybody. You never got upset and you were persistent.

Ray Vara Every morning you wake up and it's a new day, and you sort of have amnesia about what happened the day before. But that's because it was work worth doing. We also knew that there was not a tougher job in our society during this time than being a governor or mayor. We all just wanted to be supportive, which sometimes required difficult discussions.

HOW THE PANDEMIC IMPACTED COMMUNITY AND HUMAN SERVICES

Duane Kurisu, true to the founding principles of the HEC, created an old-style plantation village on former scrubland mauka of Ke'ehi Lagoon for approximately 650 formerly homeless women and their children.

Georgette Deemer I was going to ask about Kahauiki Village and what you saw for the residents there. How were they faring during the pandemic?

Duane Kurisu Throughout the pandemic, we found that the villagers were resilient people. Most never asked for handouts. However, Hawai'i people are such generous people and came forward with so many acts of kindness including Thanksgiving meals or even just individual groups and companies providing food, which they graciously took. Still, I remember going door-to-door, bringing boxes of food with some other project volunteers and some of them would say, "You know, that's okay. I think we have enough," and, "Why don't you go share with somebody else?"

Overall, the children were the ones who suffered the most. They had to do their best within the circumstances they were given. During the lockdown, they couldn't go to school and our security people, bless their souls, took responsibility on their own to be sure everyone followed the rules. Children were children, and they constantly pushed their way to go outside and play. It was especially difficult because the homes were relatively small for families. But nevertheless, security would chase them back into their homes. Some of us would need to visit the Village for maintenance purposes and the feeling was wow, because no one was visibly around. Security did their best to comply with the lockdown. Somewhat comforting was that every household was provided with high-speed internet and cable TV.

Kirk Caldwell So they didn't have any problems with online learning.

Georgette Deemer Did they have devices?

Duane Kurisu Yes, devices were donated by organizations like Kahala Clinic and aio Foundation, and the schools provided devices to those who did not already have them. Retired schoolteachers and school administrators volunteered their time to do remedial work with the children, and they would tell me that they weren't only teaching the children, they were teaching the parents too. So parents became part of the learning community.

And the learning community wasn't defined exclusively by remedial work. Villagers became teachers to other villagers. An example is a lady who started burying orange peels, apple rinds, and other organic material to create mulch. She then started growing vegetables and fruit trees. It attracted other families to want to do the same thing since the Kahauiki soil was not very good. So employees from the City donated wooden boxes and then she started teaching the families how to mulch and grow their own fruits and vegetables. The program became such an attraction that it became part of the Kahauiki Village social structure.

This could only have happened because people felt they were part of a community. It was a microcosm of people helping people. It was a testament to our core vision of building Kahauiki Village as a community rather than just being a place for shelter.

The Village has its own tenant association. It has a president, vice president, secretary, and treasurer. It is a place where families can do what they want, within normal community rules, and they can live in the Village for as long as they want.

Georgette Deemer Well, it did seem like a little microcosm of the larger community inside this little community that you were building. So it seems like a good place to get a sense of how we're doing.

Duane Kurisu Good point. We've had people from all over the world come visit. In fact, Kirk, when you hosted the United States Conference of Mayors in 2019, some of the mayors came to visit. During the tour, a number of them suggested that they intended to replicate a Kahauiki Village prototype back in their own cities. Two of them followed up with calls and surprisingly said that they couldn't do it because they didn't understand community. I remember being stunned and wondered how this could be. Has our world fallen off so badly? But then, over time, I realized what they meant was that they didn't understand community in the way they experienced during the Kahauiki Village visit. They could not replicate community in the way Hawai'i understands community. We have something really special going on here. We might consider stopping sometimes to embrace it—that which is our soul, Hawai'i's soul.

Since then, whenever I give people a tour of the Village and they see the smiling face and hear the friendly voices, I tell them that what they experience is the soul of Kahauiki Village. And that the soul of Kahauiki Village is an aggregation of the graciousness, generosity, dignity, and energy of all of the people who provided the resources for and provided the hands for building and operating Kahauiki Village. The core underlying the soul of Kahauiki Village is Hawai'i's soul. It's community building community.

Dr. David Derauf spoke about building community within one of the most vulnerable groups of O'ahu, the Pacific Islander community and the clients at Kōkua Kalihi Valley.

David Derauf (Kōkua Kalihi Valley) We should also acknowledge where we did well. Those lessons are just as important as where we faltered. And I think Hawai'i has the benefit of a group of people in society who know how to get along. Their first reaction isn't to point fingers at others. They want to take care of one another still. We have a lot of that relative to the Mainland. And yet we can see relative to some other places in the world that we don't have enough. And we should learn from that.

As an organization, our response was first and foremost driven by that concept of health as connection. What are we going to do to sustain and build those connections during a difficult time, particularly for the super high-risk kūpuna who are not just at risk for a terrible viral disease but at risk of dying of loneliness? Who's going to shop for them? Who's going to check in on them? And my coworkers here, within four days of the pandemic coming to Hawai'i, had reorganized themselves into teams to tackle that situation.

How were we able to transition like that? For about four years, we had invested heavily in building cross-department collaboration, having people work in cohorts, from across our organization, so that the dentists had gotten to know the people up here at the park. And then dental shut down. We determined we were not going to furlough people, so we had people from the dental clinic doing food runs, knocking on doors, "Auntie, how are you doing? Do you have your medicine? Can I go to Longs for you? Got enough to eat in the house? You don't have a way to do telehealth? Let's get you an iPad." I mean, everyone figured out how they could be maximally useful.

There's a lot of that in Hawai'i still, and in a community like Kalihi, there's really a lot of it. That's the one thing that has blown me away. I've been here thirty-one years in this community now, and there's a lot of people who like to talk stink about this place—the crime, the poverty—but when it comes down to it, there's a lot of "can do," too, and a lot of people who will take care of each other. We saw that in spades. Our frontline support workers doing the community food deliveries will tell you. "Hey, I grew some such and such in my yard. You like to share with the rest of the people?" Everyone wanted to be a part of doing the right thing.

One of my favorite stories, these teams would go out and they found a homeless guy living in his van and they determined he really needed a food drop, a mask, and hand sanitizer. He goes, "Nah I'm good. But can you help me fill out this form? I gotta do a job interview, but I gotta get a physical. And to get a physical, Kaiser wants me to do all this paperwork. I don't know how to do this thing."

So they took an hour, they filled out his paperwork, and thought, *I'm not sure what's going to come out of that.* But sure enough, two weeks later they're driving into public housing, he's at the guardhouse. "I got the job!"

Kirk Caldwell It just shows the barriers, that he couldn't fill out the paperwork.

David Derauf He was so excited. "I'm going to remember you every time you come through here. You're the ones who helped me get this job!"

Kirk Caldwell So the community, you say they are better. Are they stronger as a community, and are they stronger within our larger community? Are there bridges now in? Is there trust or mistrust?

David Derauf Unfortunately, dealing with the issue with our law enforcements, we have to tackle that. We have to find a forum where people can really sit down and get to know one another. I'm convinced that the beginning for this stuff is good conversation. You don't build trust overnight. Just make the effort, like bringing Shanty Asher (Pacific Island liaison for the City and County of Honolulu) on, that makes a difference. We just need more of those kinds of actions. We need the DOH to realize we've got to hire more people from that community. You've got to spend time getting to know them. They're good people.

Kirk Caldwell David, if the City and County of Honolulu had done a better job reaching out to the Pacific Islander community in the Kalihi area, would there have been a reduction in the high number of cases in that community?"

David Derauf I don't know what to make of it. And I'm going to withhold any comments until I see the next few weeks. It may be that there's enough immunity from last summer. At one point in our clinic, 35 percent of the tested were positive.

I think this community demonstrated it could pull together. So many different people came in to support us. The City was a huge support. You managed to steer support for testing initially, rental support, and all that stuff through the community health centers. That was the first time we'd ever worked together. And it was on a huge scale. And we pulled it off. It was huge. And many of our private institutions like Bank of Hawai'i, whose CEO, Peter Ho, knew it was going to take time to have stuff happen at the government level, he came to us and said, "Hey, what do you need? Tell me what you need." I was flabbergasted. To me, that's Hawai'i. That speaks to Hawai'i. Everyone says, "I have to do my part," "We could have done more on our part," "We still can do more on our part," "We still are dealing with a serious situation here. How do we figure this out?"

To me, the most important thing—the message I'm delivering to everyone is figure out how we take care of one another. Right now, what could you be doing? Your next-door neighbor, your grandma, your kid, someone you don't know—figure out how we're going to pull this off. Because we're not out of the woods. I worry because it's becoming increasingly divisive and I think there are people who would be happy to see us all at each other's throats. I don't want to see that happening in Hawai'i.

Kirk Caldwell For me, I was just blown away by so many people sacrificing so much, I think more than other places in the world. And that's part of taking care of each other, trying to do what they're asked, because it's my neighbor, my child.

David Derauf In my profession, trust is everything. You lose the trust of people and that's why I worry about every decision we make for people. I'm extremely cautious in my approach, one-on-one. People ask me if can come out and do a big event and talk to everyone in my organization. That's not how I operate. I like to get to know someone and tailor the message to that person because I know something about the risk, I know something about what will move them. Speaking to a big audience, I might just as well piss people off. *You don't know me. You don't know what you're talking about,* haole *boy.*

Kirk Caldwell Trust is everything and there's a lack of it.

IMAGINING THE FUTURE OF HAWAI'I'S VISITOR INDUSTRY

David Ige (Governor of Hawai'i) When the full brunt of the pandemic hit Hawai'i in March 2020, our number-one industry, tourism, took a dramatic hit, with arrivals dropping to historic lows with the implementation of a fourteen-day quarantine for those arriving on our shores. Our resort areas were desolate and our beaches, hiking trails, and outdoor spaces became places for residents to enjoy almost all to themselves. Even with record high unemployment resulting from those working in the visitor industry being laid off, we came to appreciate life without tourists overwhelming our natural spaces and negatively impacting our way of life. This has led to discussions at every level of government, in our business sector, and in the general public as to how to better manage our tourism industry coming out of the pandemic.

One of the people tasked with addressing this issue is John De Fries, who had just been appointed to head the HTA as the full impact of the pandemic was being felt in Hawaiʻi.

John De Fries Initially, I had wished that the legislature would have waited another year, kept the status quo at HTA, and allowed us to demonstrate what we could do from that original operating formation. It was clearly within the legislature's authority to suspend HTA's tourism special fund and terminate TAT as our sole source of funding, plus a budget reduction from $79 million to $60 million for FY22, and at the convention center budget cut from $16.5 million to $11 million for FY22. All told, these are very serious budget cuts and critical operational adjustments. Actually, I was less concerned about the budget cuts and more concerned about how the legislation would change the organizational structure and the daily operation of HTA and its contractors.

Recalling my first read of House Bill 862, I happened to be on a call with the governor and he was reading it for the first time as well. It's my nature to communicate through metaphors, so I said to the governor, "This sure feels like taking a double-hull canoe into dry dock, taking off the hulls, and putting two logs in its place, and then putting the canoe back in the water." As the governor was reading, he said in a good-spirited way, "John, at least one of the logs might be petrified." The legislation, as drafted then, would cause HTA to lose its flexibility and maneuverability, its agility and efficiency, and we would lose our responsiveness at a time when optional functionality in the economic recovery was essential.

However, in a demand for more transparency and accountability, the legislature turned HB862 to a law, which caused my staff and I to feel defeated and deflated. Subsequently, in a meeting with my leadership team, I said, "Go home this weekend and yell, scream, shout out, have a drink, punch a punching bag, do everything you can to get this negative feeling out of your system. Because Monday when you get back, you need a whole new mindset. The legislation is now the law of the land. We're going to take what we got and we're going to make it work."

Then I added, "This reminds me of my mother just putting more cabbage in the beef stew so she could feed more people. So if you see me this fiscal year walking around with cabbage, you'll understand." With the help of our entire HTA Board of Directors, our HTA leadership team and staff, we made the commitment to a changed management plan that has set a new course for HTA.

So what we did with Hawaiian programs was we went to Micah Kane at HCF, mapped out a plan that we could protect those programs for FY22, and HCF became our contractor. The other thing that we did was we contracted our foreign marketing partners, with whom we are prohibited from utilizing ARPA (federal) funds. We're on a calendar year, so their funding relative to these monies will commence in January 2022. So we were able to cover certain bases to get us through FY22.

Kirk Caldwell You were talking about conversations with the governor and the mayors. One of the things that has come out of this pandemic is more communication between the private and public sectors. For example, the visitor industry, you were on calls with all the mayors, sometimes with the governor, and you were on the VTCs (video teleconferences). I hope this doesn't go away when the pandemic goes away because I do think this kind of collaboration and bringing up issues that are problems for everyone to hear in a flat kind of management is good for everybody.

John De Fries Hawai'i was in a crisis mode before the pandemic. We have inadvertently evolved an economic model and public policies that have put future generations of kama'āina at risk of not being able to have the quality of life for things as fundamental as owning your own home or having access to affordable rental units. So we still have an array of issues to resolve, and as such, we should remain connected to bring the same intense levels of leadership that has led Hawai'i through one of the most challenging periods in modern history.

In 2019, we generated $2.2 billion in state taxes, including $600 million in TAT, so if we lose a half billion of that annual state tax revenue, where's it coming from? So if you're going to be anti-tourism, you have an opportunity to be "pro something." You as a tourism-opposition leader have the responsibility to put forth a viable alternative. Likewise, those of us who are tourism leaders need to be mindful of the fact that resident sentiments are calling for a different model of tourism.

Kirk Caldwell I had lunch with Colbert Matsumoto the other day and he was commenting on the push to diversify and get away from tourism. He opined that we've never been a diversified economy. First we had sugar, then it was sugar and pineapple and a growing military sector, and then when sugar and pineapple started declining we replaced it with tourism. We've had a few industries that have driven Hawai'i since the days of Kamehameha III. This dream that somehow we're going to get off of tourism has never really materialized. So when someone says they are against tourism, okay, what are you going to do to keep one-third of your population employed? What are they going to be doing to make a living so that they can continue to live here in Hawai'i?

John De Fries As a panelist on PBS the other night, I said, "You know, we need to start looking at tourism as a potential driver of economic diversification. Not the antithesis of diversification." As an example, I told the story about Hawai'i's culinary chefs, who thirty-plus years ago, Peter Merriman, Roy Yamaguchi, Alan Wong, Sam Choy, Bev Gannon, and Mark Ellman, to name a few, made a commitment to Hawai'i regional cuisine, and they put our Islands on the culinary map globally. And when they did that, they actually altered the way local farmers started to perceive what the visitor market might look like for their own businesses. And, so too, did the local ranchers in meat production and local fishermen, because now the quality standards had to get to the four- and five-star levels and you needed to build your capacity to meet the market demand.

Another example is to look at Hawai'i's architectural industry, which became better and more refined and sophisticated with the help of their client work in the Hawai'i hotel and resort industry, and how several Hawai'i firms began catering to resort clients around the world. Upon close examination, the tourism industry is really a composite of diversified businesses that crosses the spectrum from planning and design to IT and cybersecurity and a range of professions in between.

Kirk Caldwell That's a good point. I think the architecture firms, some of them, they're not as large as ones from the continent but they're world-class. People use them and there is a signature kind of landscape architecture and visitor industry architecture that people copy, whether it's in Singapore or China or Miami or the Bahamas. Hawai'i architects have defined a certain type of architecture and landscaping.

John De Fries Just thinking about a couple of my colleagues, like Francis Oda at Group 70 and Rob Iopa at WCIT Architecture. Awesome, homegrown, creative talent now serving both local and international clients while inspiring more local kids to enter their profession.

Georgette Deemer The pandemic also gave you the opportunity to rethink tourism. I know that even before we left, you had a plan about what tourism could look like on the other side of this whole pandemic and it was a beautiful scenario because it elevated the culture, and it decreased the number of people but increased the spending per day kind of tourist. So I was just wondering what happened to that. Is that part of your strategic plan?

John De Fries It's part of the strategic plan. It's also part of the destination management action plan (DMAP). Now every island today including O'ahu has a DMAP. Bringing together a steering committee of very diverse community members, anywhere between eighteen to twenty-four people, and in that group you could find a hotel general manager, a hotel owner, you could find a rancher, a farmer, a schoolteacher, people who were directly or indirectly affected by tourism. The more diverse the makeup of the steering committee the better.

It was also important for my staff to facilitate and remain neutral because what you want is for the people of that specific island community to envision and design a sustainable model for their community. Whatever that looks like. So the respective steering committees came together, identified the priorities, listed the hot spots where it was already problematic, and then after they put that framework together the conversation was expanded into the community for feedback and refinements.

So each DMAP has actionable items and lead agencies who are responsible for implementing the solutions for each year over a three-year period. We now have this framework in place on every island and we are working together with the island chapters of the Hawaiʻi Visitors and Convention Bureau as well as the economic development offices of each of the counties. On a quarterly basis, a progress report for each DMAP is published and made available for elected officials, industry stakeholders, and the general public to review and provide comments and new ideas.

People keep asking me, "John, don't you agree that it's time that the community be given a seat at the table?" And I respond, "Actually, it's time for all of us to recognize that the community is the table. It's their table, it's our table, and we're the hosts who invite others to sit at the table." In seeking solutions to the adverse impacts created by tourism, we must turn to the communities for help and guidance. Likewise, these communities should expect HTA and other local government agencies to find the resources required to solve these issues. Communities who live with these adverse impacts will typically have viable solutions to offer.

So the next question is, "John, what's the KPI (key performance indicator) for all these actionable items?"

Real simple. The problems, as they are identified, must be improved upon or outright resolved. That's the ultimate KPI. As a community-based program, DMAPs statewide are moving in the right direction and I've actually been extremely inspired by the intensity with which people in our communities are actually trying to understand how tourism can work.

And I'll end it with this story about Waipiʻo Valley. About every ten years, there's a flood. And the flood wipes out roads, crops, boundary lines, all that, and the community of the valley comes together and helps each other do the massive cleanup and start to rebuild and replant.

About twenty-eight years ago, I was assisting on a lease agreement project in the valley and the ten-year flood came. All of it was new to me, and in the aftermath of the flood, most people were focused on redirecting the water on the upper ridgeline of the valley to keep the excessive amounts of water from coming into the valley and help mitigate or avoid future floods.

And this Hawaiian woman, this kupuna, tells me, "John, the water is actually a gift. The problem is we don't have enough acreage under cultivation. Because if we had more *kalo*, if we had more crops and more acreage was under cultivation, this water could be channeled to where it belongs. Right now, it's just running right through the middle and all over the place causing damage." In Hawai'i tourism today, I relate to this story and the power of the metaphor. I see parallels in the manner in which the farmers of the valley manage the water flow, which in itself is innovation through the deployment of traditional practices coupled with modern technological advances.

How do we better manage the daily flow patterns of our visitors? How do we keep the visitors from over-congregating in certain places or at certain attractions at certain times of the day? Just like the waters of Waipi'o Valley, if it's not managed well each day, it can become destructive and overwhelm the well-being of the valley community. To this end, and in different parts of our state, initial steps are being taken by state and county agencies who are implementing reservations and user-fee systems.

HTA, at this time, is exploring options for a new and centralized digital infrastructure with the intent being to get real-time information to end users (local residents and visitors) that will enable them to make real-time decisions about places to visit and preferred times to make that visitation. This system would be informational, educational, culturally authentic, and transactional.

The model is called regenerative tourism. Three generations from now, the natural resources of Hawai'i have got to be in better condition than it is today. Cultural traditions three generations from now have to be thriving to a greater extent. Hawaiian language and our multiethnic traditions as a community need to be much more vibrant three generations from now. So if you and I were on a call with a hundred people right now and I said, "How many of you on the call can envision a future like that? Or would favor a vision like that?" There's no doubt in any of our minds it would be a unanimous vote in favor. And the reasons we can see that is because that's where our great-grandchildren will live and we want them to have a foundation upon which to create the quality of life they will want for themselves and the generations who will follow them.

If we can agree to that common description or vision of our future, then what is it we've got to do today in our personal lives and professional lives to put Hawaiʻi on that trajectory?

Kirk Caldwell As a kid, we went down to Waipiʻo a lot. We camped down there, we'd surf down there, we made friends with some of the Hawaiian Chinese families that grew kalo. Once, we were all down there—us five kids, my mom, my dad was working—but we got caught in one of those floods. And we had to sleep overnight on the Waimanu side of the stream. But the flood comes, the water comes fast and the water flows away pretty quickly. And it's amazing how the community comes out almost immediately rebuilding the roads through the stream, putting the stones back, getting rid of debris, restoring the *ʻauwae* that got messed up a bit. And everything starts to go to where it's supposed to go. You described a beautiful way to talk about tourism.

John De Fries The Hawaiian *ahupuaʻa* was, and remains today, a viable platform for innovation through the management of resources, human relationships, natural systems, and technological applications. As such, I actually sense that we can manage ten-plus million visitors annually, but we cannot do it with the systems that are in place today. Out of necessity and inspired by the *ahupuaʻa* system, our future in Hawaiʻi is being redesigned.

Paul Yonamine (Central Pacific Bank) ANA and Japan Airlines, they're all flying even though they have limited flights right now. But the one thing that Hawaiʻi hasn't done is to prepare for the real opening of tourism. We clearly didn't with the Mainland, but we have an opportunity to do that with Japan right now. I'm happy to report that the governor and HTA are very open, and we're working together to develop a strategy for Japan. Assuming that Japanese tourists are not coming back until January 2022, we've got four months to plan, to do better market segmentation to go after the more high-net-worth Japanese, for example, and to spend time with the airlines and talk them out of increasing their low-cost carrier strategy, which just swarms us with people who don't spend much money. We have an opportunity to make improvements. I've been talking to the governor about organizing strategy so that as soon as Japan lifts the fourteen-day quarantine, we will be the first to market travel in Japan. That means millions of dollars of free media coverage and everybody there wants to come here anyway. We have to exploit and capitalize those opportunities. Nobody here was taking the lead on that strategy, so that's my focus right now. We're trying to make plans for that eventuality of an influx in Japanese tourism.

Kirk Caldwell And John De Fries, of HTA, would have to reach out that way too.

Paul Yonamine We missed the opportunity to redefine tourism. John came in and said Malama Hawai'i, which I personally thought was great. Let's come up with a new cultural spiritual concept of Hawai'i tourism. It would allow us to go after interested tourists because they're likely the ones who are going to spend more money anyway. But you need to have a strategic plan and to be able to execute off of, which we didn't have with the US Mainland. We do have that opportunity now with Japan, so aside from my banking time, I'm collaborating on that.

Georgette Deemer It must be a little scary, though, because the local response to tourism is so negative right now and they're saying, "If it's this bad now and Asia has not even arrived yet..."

Paul Yonamine I think that's why it's important for leadership to have a vision of the future of tourism in Hawai'i. What if it's five million people a year, but we triple the individual spend? But we don't yet have a strategy to accomplish that. Local venues could change to become more cultural and spiritual, but you can't bring a Target customer to a Louis Vuitton store and expect them to start buying high-end products. You have to match the customer with what you're selling. So far, we have been very insular in our approach. We try to fix things here in Hawai'i without regard for the customer, which right now is the Japanese tourist. We need to market to the right people and we can do that with data and digital marketing, but it takes a lot of political will. You need leadership willing to drive that strategy.

Kirk Caldwell I was hoping that was going to happen under the governor's leadership. I don't know if we've lost the opportunity. I still think there's opportunity there to try to reconfigure because there's so much pushback. I think it's going to continue and get worse.

Paul Yonamine Again, it's so hard. I'm not in the governor's shoes and he's got to deal with COVID. David's a really nice guy. He wants to make sure nobody dies. That's his top issue. Perhaps there are people around him who should have been thinking more about economic development post-COVID. But I don't think that change is a lost opportunity. We have time to do something with Japan, to create a case study, a reference point that we can apply to other major departure locations, and see where we go from there. We're giving it a stab right now. It's amazing, for example, that the State of Hawai'i has no data on visitors that's readily available to use for offshore marketing.

The Department of Agriculture has data, but they won't let us use it. There's data in other parts of the state, but it's blocked by concerns with privacy. A lot of the people who filled in the survey data didn't give us permission to use it for marketing, so the attorney general won't release it. Where does that put us today? We're in data collection—we're starting from zero.

Previously, I started the Hawai'i campaign for McDonald's Japan with Eric Takahata of Hawaii Tourism Japan. We collected data on half a million Japanese citizens. We know income levels and everything, and we can't use any of it. The State will not allow us to use it.

Kirk Caldwell I agree, the governor is a good guy. I told him once in a meeting in his cabinet room how upset I was with him, and even more upset that despite this fact, I really liked him. Why? Because he is smart, reads everything, and wants to do the right thing. In the end, he wants to protect all of us. It is just that he is very slow in making decisions.

Paul Yonamine There is a need to delegate more and empower more. Sometimes there's delegation but there's no empowerment. Then you're a lame duck. The jury's out about how the governor has handled the pandemic. He has faced a lot of criticism, but at the end of the day it is true that Hawai'i is one of the safest states in the nation, and so I think that when things finally settle, we'll reflect back and maybe find that what he did was spot on. I don't know. I even told him that I might have been overly critical of him. We are, today, a relatively safe community as a result of his decisions. But then again, we sure as heck worried a lot, and I did debrief him about that. Good leaders help people gain confidence so they don't have to waste their time getting all stressed out and worried. To that end, I think he could have done a better job of making us feel more confident about our course. If they feel capable, people spend time more productively by looking for new answers, solutions, and strategies.

I think he possibly could have done a better job at empowerment, but in terms of protecting us, he might have nailed it.

Kirk Caldwell And he didn't waver. He showed leadership and stood his ground.

Paul Yonamine I think you did too, Kirk, with your tier system. Was that perfect? Absolutely not, but it was a guideline. People needed it. We can debate and refine the structure, but at least you had something in place when it was needed.

Almost all the frontline leaders we interviewed believed that our responses to the pandemic were unique from the rest of the country and perhaps the world. They felt it is something we should be proud of. There also were missed opportunities. Most felt it was the most challenging issue of their professional lives.

David Ige (Governor of Hawai'i) For me, I think that Hawai'i should be proud of the COVID response. All of the community came together. And obviously there are some that have to make decisions on behalf of the community, but we knew that there would be support at the end. That's what makes Hawai'i such a special place.

Mike Victorino (Mayor of Maui County) I really can't speak for those in other places, but I can say in Hawai'i, whatever the challenge comes forth, we band together as a community to do what we can to protect the well-being of our citizens, our families, and friends. So I feel very confident we've always been resilient. We know we're 2,500 miles away from any landmass and there's not another state that's going to drive in or take a train into our county and help us. So we know outside help will take days, if not weeks to come. So we have to take care of our own community. I believe Maui County, like the rest of the state, has done a really terrific job overall. All of the mayors, all of the medical staff, their executive teams, communities, nonprofits, business, as well as our state government, in general, has really had a warm heart and really tried their best to take care of the needs of the people of our state and our counties.

COVID'S IMPACT ON EDUCATION

Christina Kishimoto I had more feedback from the governor. I felt like I reported to the governor this whole year. And I don't report to the governor, but rather to the Board of Education. But I appreciate that he was there and answered all of my calls. I appreciated that he asked, "What do you want to do?" and he was a sounding board. And several times I would ask him, "Do you think you can call the mayors together? I'd like to talk to them. I don't want them surprised about what I'm thinking." And he'd say, "Yep, this meeting is coming up. I'm going to add you to the agenda," or "I'm going to call this meeting." That's what

I needed. Help like that. And that was helpful. Kirk, you and I talked a couple of times. Whether it was about graduation or how you were thinking about tiering and how many people can gather and masking, that was helpful to be able to just call you. We had these strange rules about when I could talk to the board, or not talk to them, and we didn't talk. I went from a board that really was locked arm in arm with me for three years, to a year of... we had changes in the board members. The board that's there now is not the board that hired me four years ago, and we know that often happens with superintendents.

Tim Cottrell (ʻIolani School) We did pretty well. We were held up as one of the models nationally, and we've been in a lot of national press about being able to do this. We're fortunate to have a community that enabled us to safely have the whole school year back on campus for all grades in a noncontroversial way. We took it super seriously and were able to do it.

I think our community in general in the state of Hawaiʻi is less divided because we're less politically divided. I think we were shielded from much of the hateful divisive politics that were going on in the Mainland and we were able to keep more cohesiveness here. I think that made us different as a place. I think public education here probably looked very much like public education in California or anywhere else. Nothing could be put into place to manage how large the system was to get kids back.

Independent schools, like ʻIolani, all of them are self-selecting communities, so we do well, but we also have families that buy into what we do. So that is very different from public education. Public education has a very heterogeneous group of people. Some families are doing great; some families are living in poverty; they have different backgrounds, values, and realities. It would be hard to get the uniformity of everybody at home saying, "Did you wear your face mask correctly today?" And here, I can say, "Parents, please ask your child and make sure they wear their face mask correctly." That's a huge benefit. Our scale is much smaller and our communities are more homogeneous.

For more than ten years now, we've also had a program called KAʻI that works closely with hundreds of families in Pālolo Valley. Leaders interviewed for this book had the challenges for those families and their students in public schools, we worked closely with them to ensure they were cared for during the pandemic. We provided all of our KAʻI students with cellular-enabled iPads, hosted several food drives that also enabled us to keep our Sodexo staff employed, provided rental assistance when needed, and online tutoring support to ensure that our KAʻI students were supported.

Georgette Deemer How many boarders do you have? Were they able to go home at all?

Tim Cottrell It was a mixed bag. In 2020, we had to have everybody leave because we closed the school. And we also had to place students who couldn't leave with families around here. Some kids left, some kids were here for two years without getting back home. So we placed them. Last year we had about seventy-five kids in the program, and maybe thirty of them were online, almost all of those students being from China, and that was just, well, there were two things happening. The whole visa process got messed up because of the federal government's position on visas. Without a pandemic, that was getting messed up anyway. And then everybody had their own quarantine issues. So, if you were a child here who lived in China—say you lived in Wuhan and you're trying to get home—okay, from here you can't fly directly to China because the government stopped, both governments had problems there. So you'd go to Vietnam or you'd go to Korea and then you'd have to do two weeks there in quarantine. Then you'd go to China and you'd have to do two weeks there. It was like a month of quarantine, so the students didn't do that. Last year, they stayed home. And then this year, we had maybe a little over a hundred kids in the program. It's bounced back really strong from all over the world and we're not doing anything online. They're all showing up.

It's complicated. You can imagine the complications of being in a dorm if somebody's positive. But again, we emphasize being vaccinated. Also, because we oversee their social lives, our boarding students are actually less exposed than the kid who's going to the beach with their friends and getting into a car with a bunch of other kids. We've kind of got them in a protected space and we can test them as much as we need to. The dorm students right now are also tested twice a week. Everybody gets tested twice a week. Just to make sure nothing spins up within the vaccinated kids.

Kirk Caldwell You've done a great job. That's why we wanted to interview you.

Tim Cottrell Well, the other part that made it work—the whole one-team ethos at ʻIolani helped tremendously. We have a culture that is about working together and taking care of each other. I think that helped us be successful all along the way.

COVID'S IMPACT ON MANAGING HEALTHCARE

Mark Mugiishi (HMSA) One of the things that happened in Hawaiʻi in spite of the fits and starts and all these little regrets, when we say in general that we did well, it was because a lot of people came together for a common goal. And so, as an old coach, that's what I used to preach. You gotta have one team, one goal, put aside your ego, and let's do this together. That was really front and center. That was a big life lesson.

We talked about public-private partnerships, community-based public-private partnerships, like HEC tries to do. They're the wave of the future. You have to if you're going to do big things.

In Hawaiʻi, we are more compliant as a group. You know, I walk around and 20 percent of the people don't have masks. Let me tell you, it's the opposite and flipped in other places—only 20 percent of the people are wearing masks. I think that's because people here care a little bit more about social responsibility. They care about ʻohana. The statements like "Do this or that, you're protecting your neighbors," has more meaning here than in many other places, and I think that was important also. You're not going to get everybody with that message but a lot more than in many other places.

Jonathan Dworkin (Queen's Health System) There are two major things. One is the history of epidemic disease in Hawai'i and the tragedy of what happened to the Hawaiian people. I don't think you can talk about the pandemic without acknowledging that the whole creation of the Queen's Medical Center happened in the shadow of a devastating epidemic disease that depopulated the Hawaiian Islands and destroyed the Hawaiian people.

For me as an ID [infectious disease] doc walking around in early 2020, I'm walking through Queen's Hospital, which was built in the wake of a smallpox epidemic, and I'm looking up at the portrait of Queen Emma on the wall, and I'm thinking to myself, *Boy, I gotta step up. This is, historically, the cause of great tragedy here and we have to do everything we can to make sure that this history doesn't repeat itself here in Hawai'i.* And you can find parallels of the native peoples on the Mainland for that, but there's something very unique about Hawai'i and in particular with Queen's.

The other big thing is because we're an island state, you can really lean into the geography of the islands and use that as a way of keeping the pandemic at bay. And I started having those thoughts early on, but they kind of came to maturation around the time we produced those letters and the Safe Travels program began. Then some of us wanted to see a stronger version of the Safe Travels program with the second post-arrival test. But using the island geography to protect the population of the island from the pandemic is a big difference between us and other places. To the extent that we were able to lean into the geography and use that as one of our tools, I think that's one of the reasons why we were successful. So, initially, the fourteen-day quarantine, and then the prearrival testing, and then the various county modifications on the prearrival testing made a huge difference. I think those are all important things.

Libby Char (Hawai'i DOH) I think our experience is in many ways the same as other places, but I think we have some unique factors as well. We're an island state and our geography is unique. We have a natural border so it creates challenges, but we should also take advantage of it. Second is that the counties are all separated and so that's made a difference in terms of things that we're trying to do at a state level. You must take into account that there are significant differences county to county. Third, our cultural background has actually lent itself to our population doing a really good job. We have much better mask compliance than many places on the Mainland. People in Asia have been wearing masks for years and years and I think that influence has made it more acceptable here. We have a better sense of community in Hawai'i—doing things for the good of the community rather than for you as an individual. That makes this a wonderful and special place to live.

TEST OF LEADERSHIP

Kirk Caldwell Was this pandemic the most difficult challenge you've encountered in your professional life?

Micah Kane (Hawai'i Community Foundation) Yeah, I would say so. Most complex, but also invigorating. One of the most invigorating experiences of my life. Our team became so much closer. We're all little microcosms of our community and we grew a lot as a team here. A lot of the little internal nuances that we talk about in our community we had in our own organization. We're a way stronger team today than we ever were and we are trying to make sure that we build on that. It was just everybody being vulnerable. It was emotional because we felt very proximate to the people we were helping. Getting intel from the nonprofits.

We normally serve as an intermediary, so we're one step removed from really seeing the people we're serving. This put us right in front of them, so it was an emotional journey for us.

Ron Mizutani (Hawai'i Foodbank) The topic of sustainability really has to come into play post-pandemic because we need to be able to be self-sustaining in some way. During Iniki's recovery, people on Kaua'i, that's why I talk about roughing it, they understood you're not going to sit there and have the same kind of meal you had every night, pre-Iniki. *I'm just here to survive and whatever calorie intake that takes*—sometimes it's just spam and rice, sometimes it's not even that. But people learn to make do with what they have. And that's what a real crisis would take. People would have to really think about how they give nutrition to their bodies just to move on until help can arrive.

This COVID crisis has really taught us a lot about our shortfalls, not only professionally but also individually. But at the same time, it also showed us how great a state we live in and when push comes to shove, we'll be there for each other. I still feel that way even though we're still fighting this thing every day.

In the end, we think Derek Kawakami, the mayor of Kaua'i County, the smallest of the counties in terms of landmass and population, but the oldest in terms of geological history, said it best. He brings it down to a very human level and gives people hope.

Derek Kawakami Yeah, well, you know, I've been in a place in my life where I had lost hope. I've been pretty public about being completely alcohol-free going on almost two and a half years. Alcoholism and addiction run in our DNA, in my family, unfortunately, and I got to a point in my life where it just seemed so hard to get the ship back on course. A lot of people won't understand and think that I have a perfect life. In many cases I'm blessed, but I'm also blessed that I was able to deal with addiction. Here I am as an elected official and as an alcoholic right at the beginning of me becoming mayor. It became clear that I could really be a great mayor or a really junk one, and it's pretty much one thing.

I've always had a strong mind and once I put my mind to something, which takes a while sometimes, but once I put my mind to something and I make a commitment, I have a high level of confidence that I will succeed. I feel that there are many people in our community that are just like me. They have a despair, they're living in a sort of darkness. Like I said before, fear is a very strong emotion. And at that time, I said, "Right now, what our little island needs, they need a vulnerable mayor that's going to let the people know that I'm just as flawed as everybody else, dealing with the same things." That in and of itself gives people a sense of hope.

With that background, maybe I'm not that bad. Social media is something that can be addressed. We wanted to do that, but you never really know how people are responding to it. But we've had a few people say that we really helped them get through some real tough times. Those are the moments that I live for. You know and I know, we're just in this to help people.

Kirk Caldwell Something that was missing during the early days of the pandemic was a sense of hope. Very few leaders were projecting that. You were, by making yourself vulnerable.

Derek Kawakami Well, I'll tell you this. If I was still dealing with alcohol during this pandemic, a lot more people would have gotten really sick and probably died. Everything happens for a reason. As my mom always said, "Pray." She would instill a deep sense of faith in us, and she'd always say things happen for a reason. And when I look back, making a commitment to stay away from the bottle, and the pandemic hitting, and being able to get through a pandemic and not touch the bottle, and have that yearning—all these things are happening to me for a reason. I think that's why I embrace it. That's why people ask me, "How do you deal with it?" And I'm like, "I'm just dealing with it like everybody else." I don't think of it as a negative thing. I think of it as what's happening and, in some way, it's going to be better for me. It's going to make me better. That's how I look at it.

Kirk Caldwell Derek, you are one of the most authentic politcians I've ever met. It's reaffirming. Honesty and being real is an attractive thing.

Derek Kawakami It's the best thing we can do, exposing our vulnerability, because that's the only way we can normalize the conversation. I remember Micah Kane came up real early in my term as mayor. I had lost my mom, eighteen months later I lost my dad, and six months after that I lost my older brother to suicide. Micah Kane came, as he does to every island, to find out from the leaders what the most pressing need was. [Hawai'i senate president Ron] Kouchi had told him we're concerned about suicide on Kaua'i, our numbers are a little higher than the statewide average. So Micah comes in and says, "Before I start, usually we go around the table, but I got a call from the senate president and he said that suicide is a big thing." It was still fresh and everybody on Kaua'i knows that I lost my brother, so the whole table just went ice cold. Nobody said anything. It was awkward.

I said, "My brother committed suicide and I'm not uncomfortable talking about it." In fact, I talk about it quite a bit now because I don't want somebody else to have to deal with the lifelong questioning of who, why, could I have done more—and that's when it becomes about just letting people know, no be shame. You're not going to solve anything by brushing it under the rug. Let's normalize the conversation.

Just gotta be real. My mom would say, "Son, you're not everybody's cup of tea and never will be, so just be your own cup of tea and be happy with yourself." I've always felt comfortable in my own skin, with my weird kinks, and I know not everybody's going to get me.

As far as our history, I think the takeaway is—and it goes back to this. My first day at work as mayor, I woke up like any other newly elected, sworn in mayor and wondered, *What the hell am I supposed to do?* I remember saying to my wife that first day, "I don't know what the hell I'm supposed to do. There was no orientation. Nobody told me. Do I report straight to the office or do I go to the civic center and the DMV? There's no handbook." And she said, "Go write one." And, you know, in this sense I think for any big challenge—I learned a lot from my mom and dad, and I learned a lot from my wife—who I am today is a collective experiment of the many people that have molded me.

My dad would always tell me true leaders wait for the opportunity. Where like any prize fighter, they want to fight the best they can to see where they stand when they are tested. Because we have all these questions. *Am I going to be able to perform under pressure? Am I going to be able to make the decisions, the important decisions in the appropriate manner?* I had all those questions in my head. And I remember my dad always telling me I have windows of opportunity. Those are the times where you can answer those questions in your head. *Am I good enough? Am I strong enough? Am I smart enough?* It will come by every day and when they do you better be ready to identify them and you better be ready to step up because it may never come back again. The last thing you want is to live a life of having those questions in your head and not having them answered.

So here we are writing a book dealing with a big, challenging situation and in a sense all of us are really blessed that we've had this opportunity to be tested on one of the greatest challenges that I think I'll know in my lifetime, so far, and still every day is the same. We wake up, we put on our shoes. We're like everybody else out there. We have the same fears. We probably have the same insecurities. But if we do things right, we rise to the challenge and I'm very thankful, Mayor. *

EPILOGUE

Where Do We Go from Here?

When we started conducting the interviews for this book, we thought we were writing a book that would be published just as the COVID pandemic came to an end. Little did we know that while our administration dealt with two surges in 2020, at a time when there were no vaccines and few effective treatment protocols for COVID, that there would be a Delta surge and an Omicron surge in the year after we left the Hale. Who knows when COVID will be swept from our shores forever? Perhaps there will never be a finish line for this virus. Yet here is what we learned from interviewing the decision makers in this book.

NO ONE IS SAFE UNTIL WE ARE ALL SAFE

There is a danger in declaring the pandemic is over. As the state, country, and world crawl out of the rubble of this pandemic, we cannot forget that our common fate matters. COVID-19 originated in Wuhan, China; the Delta variant came from a mutation in India; and the Omicron variant came from a mutation in South Africa. Variants will emerge even if we try to put the past behind us and forget the lessons learned from this worldwide pandemic. No one is truly safe until we are all safe.

Hawai'i is the most isolated group of islands from any other landmass in the world. But one lesson we should have learned from this pandemic is that despite this geographic isolation, we remain connected to everywhere else. Unless we build a wall around our islands, use the Pacific Ocean as a moat, and prohibit people from entering or leaving our state, we will remain susceptible to viruses and future pandemics.

In the interest of self-preservation, we must work to support the building of the infrastructure to get the rest of the world, particularly the least developed parts of our world, fully vaccinated and boosted to protect against COVID-19 and its variants. Not only because of our own interest in self-preservation, but also because it is the right thing to do. If there is one thing that the people of Hawaiʻi understand it is the nature of *kuleana* and our shared responsibility.

THE STRUCTURE FOR FIGHTING FUTURE PANDEMICS

We also have been told that with a rapidly warming planet and the resulting acceleration of our climate crisis around the globe, we can expect to see more worldwide pandemics. So now is not the time to let our guard down and, perhaps more importantly, to forget the lessons learned from the current COVID pandemic, lest we repeat the same mistakes again. We also must ask ourselves, Are we willing to think in the long term and commit to a long-term plan of action? In short, how can Hawaiʻi successfully navigate future pandemics?

There is little doubt that through the last two and half years we have developed a strong COVID muscle through our shared experience in Hawaiʻi. We do not want it to atrophy. This means we must continue to exercise this muscle, and for lack of a better word, develop "muscle memory."

A group of publicly minded and strongly committed people have been meeting over the prior year and authored a paper titled "Kiaʻi—Guarding Hawaiʻi From Future Outbreaks: Lessons Learned from the COVID-19 Pandemic in Hawaiʻi, 2020–2022." The authors are Jonathan Dworkin, Michael Schwartz, Kapono Chong-Hanssen, Lee Altenberg, Darragh O'Carroll, Robert Weiner, and Lee Evslin. As seen in the chapters preceding this one, Dr. Dworkin was in the mayor's advisory group on COVID-19 and a major influence in getting the City and County of Honolulu to take a more proactive and action-oriented approach to controlling the spread of COVID-19. Dr. O'Carroll was instrumental in the early days of the pandemic in helping the City and County of Honolulu roll out a vigorous face covering program, along with working with communities of need in protecting themselves from the spread of COVID-19. They have developed a road map for ensuring that Hawai'i is better prepared for the next pandemic when it arrives on our shores. We have adopted many of their recommendations and added others that are lifted from the chapters of this book.

WHERE DOES THE DECISION-MAKING PROCESS RESIDE?

The first question that needs to be answered is what entity or entities, government or nongovernment, should lead the response to a pandemic? From our experience during the first year of the pandemic, it is our conclusion that the DOH is ill-equipped to lead the response to a statewide health crisis such as the COVID-19 pandemic. Maybe no state health department can successfully carry out such a response. We have seen the numerous failures in other states across our nation and we have seen a record number of health directors from these states either resign or be fired because of mistakes made in responding to the pandemic. Sometimes they were just relying on the best scientific information and medical advice available at the time. It was not always their fault.

Yet there is something in the structure of health departments that prevent them from not only responding quickly, but also quickly implementing the actions that need to be taken to address the devastating impacts of widespread natural disasters such as pandemics. That response more commonly resides with emergency management agencies on the federal, state, and county level. And for the most part, these agencies are better able to address the impacts of emergencies such as hurricanes, floods, tsunamis, forest and brush fires, earthquakes, and other natural disasters.

Our conclusion, therefore, is that the response to a pandemic should lie with the emergency response agencies. Because we do not want to leave our fate up to the advice of federal agencies given what occurred under the Trump administration, we need to bring it home to Hawai'i and place it squarely under Hawai'i's Emergency Management Agency (HI-EMA). The DOH should be placed in the lead advisory role. Each of the four county emergency management agencies must be equal copartners with HI-EMA because of the statewide nature of a pandemic and because the counties are where the implementation of the pandemic response will be carried out through their large and embedded police, fire, and emergency management functions and personnel. The Hawai'i National Guard would assist through HI-EMA.

Science, public health, and evidence-based medical advice must be at the core of every decision made in responding to a pandemic. As is evident from the chapters of this book, it is ill-advised to base this responsibility solely with the DOH. As the COVID-19 pandemic unfolded, we witnessed the organic formation of medical panels, such as the one put together by the City and County of Honolulu, those hosted by the Hawai'i Executive Collaborative, and the Hawai'i State Senate and House committees on COVID-19. It is critical that input is received from the private medical and public health sectors, and not just from the government sector led by the DOH.

The presidents and CEOs of the largest healthcare systems, the largest health insurance provider, practicing physicians from these healthcare systems, and community healthcare systems from all counties, along with professors and others from the University of Hawai'i system, including the John A. Burns School of Medicine, must be placed at the same table as the director of the DOH to provide real-time advice on actions that need to be taken to control the outbreak and spread of any virus.

While not directly related to public health and safety, Hawai'i's education system, both public and private, was left woefully out of the discussions when decisions were made regarding the COVID-19 pandemic, and this had a significant impact on the educational and social health of our children and young adults. This cannot be allowed to happen again. The superintendent of education, the president of the University of Hawai'i, and the head of the Hawaii Association of Independent Schools also must be at the table and have direct input into the decisions being made.

Of equal importance is the input of Hawai'i's multifaceted business community regarding how proposed actions and responses will impact their business and how best to mitigate that impact where possible.

This group would include leaders from our visitor industry; the heads of major corporations; and not-for-profits such as the Hawai'i Community Foundation, the Hawai'i Executive Collaborative, the Hawaii Business Roundtable, Chamber of Commerce Hawai'i, and the Hawai'i Restaurant Association, among other entities. As you will recall some of these individuals were the most proactive in responding to the growing COVID-19 pandemic and were way out in front of the DOH in actions that needed to be taken to protect the people of Hawai'i.

While this is a large group of people, they all should have a seat at the table to share information, to hear the debates and discussions, and to have an equal say in what actions need to be taken. The final decisions on how to respond and what actions are to be taken reside with the executive branch of the state and county governments.

THE SHARING OF DATA AND TRANSPARENCY IS CRITICAL TO SUCCESSFULLY MANAGE THE SPREAD OF A VIRUS DURING A PANDEMIC.

To ensure the most successful outcomes, there must be a sharing of data, open analysis of the data, and transparency with the public. Emergency management agencies and the DOH in non-pandemic situations are set up to preserve privacy and protect confidential information. Therefore, there could be pushback from government officials and others to include such a large gathering of individuals in meetings and discussions on responding to the next pandemic. This must be met with the reality that the sharing of such information and transparency is vital for a successful pandemic response. Demographic and epidemiological data should be shared between entities and these entities should not prevent the sharing of pertinent information claiming that they "own" such data. In a pandemic crisis, helpful data should be shared. This should include mobile phone software that can be used to provide the population with reliable, up-to-date information. The public must know where the virus is spreading in real time, so it knows where to avoid gathering. This is important for promoting trust and confidence in the government response.

FRAMEWORK

What follows is a suggested framework to put in place to successfully address this and future pandemics. This framework comes out of our shared experience as described in the chapters of this book and from the article, "Kia'i—Guarding Hawai'i from Future Outbreaks," referenced previously.

TRAVEL RESTRICTIONS AND TESTING

Our best defense to protect Hawaii from a pandemic that is spreading around the globe is to take advantage of our geographic isolation, which greatly enables our ability to restrict movement across our borders. The fourteen-day quarantine put in place by Governor Ige was effective in reducing the spread of COVID-19. With the loosening of these restrictions in October 2020, we saw a resulting increase in transmission of the virus. A quarantine mandate should be kept as one of the most effective tools in controlling the spread of a virus. Exemptions to a quarantine mandate should be kept to a minimum, including exemptions for military personnel stationed in Hawai'i.

Post-arrival testing, regardless of symptoms, can be an effective tool to evaluate the impact of reopening our borders. There should be hotels on contract to isolate those who test positive for the pathogen. The State should also ensure that rapid antigen tests be readily available to conduct post-arrival testing. Contracts for such tests should be in place prior to a virus arriving on our shores.

TESTING, TRACING, AND ISOLATION FACILITIES

The City and County of Honolulu was an early supporter for 1) increasing testing capacity for its residents, 2) making sure we had sufficient contact tracers for those residents who tested positive for COVID and those who came into close contact with such individuals, and 3) having sufficient isolation facilities for individuals who could not safely isolate at home. Prior to Dr. Libby Char becoming the director of the

DOH, the City and County was not supported in these efforts, which forced the City to go it alone. This cannot be repeated again, as these three legs of the stool are critical in controlling and then containing the spread of a pathogen.

This capacity must be developed locally and the structure should be in place for building out such capacity well before a virus reaches our shores. Central coordination of these resources is essential and it makes sense that HI-EMA be the coordinating authority, with resources from the Hawai'i National Guard and the four county mayors. The DOH would be the lead agency in advising on the appropriate testing methods and the protocols for contact tracing, and it would have the management responsibility of the isolation sites. We cannot emphasize enough the importance of successfully integrating these three critical elements into any pandemic response.

MASKS AND PPE

Masks and PPE are equally low-cost interventions to fighting a pathogen. Early implementation of a universal masking policy will slow the spread of most viruses. Surgical masks are more effective than cloth masks. HI-EMA should be tasked with locating and maintaining access to a strategic stockpile of N95 masks and PPE that can be readily distributed prior to a pathogen reaching Hawai'i's shores.

MEDICATIONS, OXYGEN, AND VACCINES

As we saw in dealing with COVID-19, medications, oxygen, and vaccines were lifesavers for those who fell sick from the virus. HI-EMA, in coordination with the Healthcare Association of Hawaii and Hawai'i's private healthcare system, should make sure that there is an effective system to obtain and distribute critical medications, including antiviral medications and oxygen for all our hospitals, public and private, and other healthcare providers where appropriate.

Hawai'i's vaccine rollout was very effective compared to other parts of the country. Both the state government and the county governments along with our private healthcare system really stepped up in developing a system for distributing the vaccines and then rolling out the vaccine program for the residents of the state of Hawai'i. This program and distribution system and all of its components should be memorialized for use in inoculating our population against the next variant or virus to appear in Hawai'i.

Vaccine mandates are effective in working towards herd immunity and should be considered when fighting future viruses. However, a non-judgmental and respectful tone should be used toward vaccine hesitant residents whenever possible. A sense of unity, that we are one community, will help to get more residents protected rather than digging in and creating even greater divisiveness on the issue of vaccinations.

We must not forget rural and underserved communities when dealing with all three of these issues of medications, oxygen, and vaccines.

EDUCATION

As is clear from this book, public education was left out in the cold and pretty much had to fend for itself during the COVID-19 pandemic, except for last-minute "lifesaving" actions by Governor Ige. Hawai'i's children suffered tremendously as a result. The private school system seemed to manage better, because of its smaller student population and an ability to work through bureaucracies better. Schools are essential both socially and economically. If we were to revise our reopening strategy, schools would be prioritized in a way that recognizes education as equal to the economy.

The governor needs to ensure that the children of Hawai'i have all the support needed to attend school. The administration must eliminate any institutional or political obstacles to making schools safe and returning our children to in-person classroom learning as soon as possible. During times of distance learning, there must be access to Wi-Fi and distribution of digital devices to any children who need them. During a pandemic crisis, the legislature should not stand in the way of the governor, but instead team up with the executive branch to make sure the children of our public school system get all that is required to keep them learning and thriving emotionally, psychologically, and academically.

STEPPING FORWARD TOGETHER

Books like this usually end with a conclusion, but we don't believe that there will be a conclusion to the pandemic in the near future. What we can take away from this experience is that strong leadership is the key to protecting our population, our economy, and our ability to recover for the future.

The leaders interviewed for this book had the following traits in common.

1. They were not afraid to make decisions, even if there was a strong chance that they could be wrong. In a pandemic, it's more important to act quickly. Lives were and still are at stake.

2. If needed, they maintained humility to admit their mistakes and correct the course.

3. They believe that working together and sharing information, even with their fiercest competitors, is the right thing to do in a pandemic. The results are more rewarding for everyone.

4. During a pandemic, they believe, it might be necessary to break old rules and make new ones. If the old rules don't work or apply to the situation, leaders must understand the need to change them.

5. They recognized the opportunity to become something better than pre-pandemic norms. Some even felt that it would be

impossible to go back to any kind of normalcy. We find that exciting.

6. They agree that Hawaiʻi is a unique place. Our people come together to form a unique community. And what we've always described as the aloha spirit, however one defines it, became evident in our response to the pandemic.

We want to thank the leaders who took the time to be interviewed, to share their wisdom, and to open their hearts and minds on what may be the most damaging health and economic crisis in our lives. They all pointed out that there was no playbook, no instructions on how to respond to a global pandemic, and that in itself highlighted the importance for them to contribute to this project. We plan to donate any profits from the sale of this book to the John A. Burns School of Medicine, and request that if possible, we would like to see greater support for a public health curriculum. If we can collectively help future generations to preserve and strengthen our beloved home of Hawaiʻi, it would be our great privilege. ❋

About the Authors

Kirk Caldwell served as mayor of the City and County of Honolulu for eight years, terming out at the end of 2020. The COVID-19 response became the first priority during the last year of his administration, when he worked side by side with Hawai'i's top leaders—none of whom had a playbook for managing a deadly pandemic. He saw the need to document, for future leaders, how Honolulu and the state of Hawai'i quickly became one of the safest places in the world. Caldwell has been an attorney for much of his career and was managing partner of a large Honolulu law firm before running for public office. He has also served as majority leader in the Hawai'i State House of Representatives and as city managing director. He continues to pursue his love for public service.

Georgette Takushi Deemer served as deputy managing director for the City and County of Honolulu during the Caldwell administration. Her professional background is in communications, and she was previously communications director for the Hawai'i State House of Representatives, as well as the Hawai'i state film commissioner, bringing television and motion picture production to the Islands and overseeing construction of the Hawai'i Film Studio at Diamond Head.